THE

MIGRAINE DIET

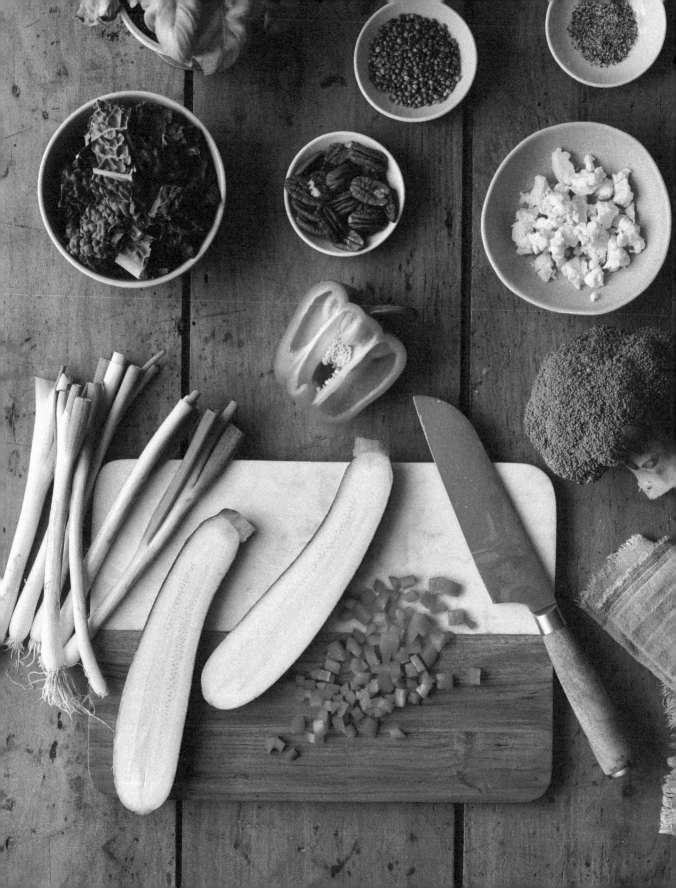

THE

MIGRAINE DIET

A Ketogenic Meal Plan
for Headache Relief

DENISE POTTER, RDN, CSP, CDE

ROCKRIDGE
PRESS

For general information on our other products and services or to obtain technical support, please contact our Customer Care Department within the U.S. at (866) 744-2665, or outside the U.S. at (510) 253-0500.

Rockridge Press publishes its books in a variety of electronic and print formats. Some content that appears in print may not be available in electronic books, and vice versa.

Interior and Cover Designer: Peatra Jariya
Photo Art Director/Art Manager: Janice Ackerman
Editor: Michael Goodman
Production Editor: Chris Gage
Photography: © 2019 Darren Muir. Food Styling by Yolanda Muir. Interior Photography Darren Muir, except on following pages: p. 2: Nadine Greeff; p. 14: Thomas J. Story; p. 24: Nadine Greeff; p. 81: Thomas J. Story; p. 195: Thomas J. Story.

ISBN: Print 978-1-64152-961-7 | eBook 978-1-64152-962-4
R0

TO MY FAVORITE HUSBAND
AND FOUR AWESOME KIDS.
I TRULY APPRECIATE
ALL OF YOUR SUPPORT.

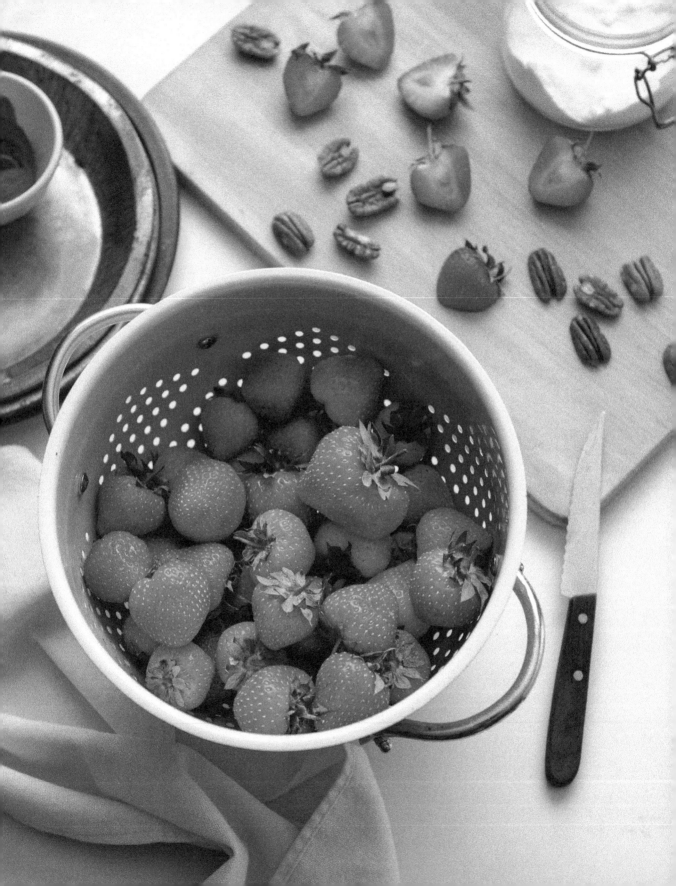

CONTENTS

INTRODUCTION

MIGRAINE. It can mean several things. Migraine might mean you aren't able to go to work today. It might mean you're going to be fired for taking too many sick days. For me, it brings back memories of huddling in a dark bedroom, wishing it would somehow just stop. It means standing over the trash can in my office at work, vomiting after an especially stressful day. It means, "I hope I can drive home today because I really can't see—there are blank spots in my vision. Oh yeah, and I can't seem to read either . . . words keep disappearing from the page."

. . . .

If you have migraines, you know *exactly* what I mean. And since you have found your way to this book, I assume your plight is not over and you're seeking a solution—or better yet, a cure.

You're not alone if you haven't been able to cure your migraines, or even get them to a tolerable level. According to the American Migraine Foundation, migraines affect more than 37 million men, women, and children in the United States alone—one out of every 11 people. And 30 percent of women will be affected by migraines over the course of their lifetime.

If this condition responded well to treatment, everyone would just take a pill and go on their merry way. But it doesn't work like that, does it? To treat migraines we turn to medication, meditation, lifestyle and dietary modifications, holistic therapies, alternative medicine, and exercise. Yet here we are, with millions still suffering when there really is hope.

I am truly excited to offer this book as a solution for many of you. While traditional treatments offer relief to some, none can offer a cure. The change in diet and lifestyle presented here, using a ketogenic diet, has been shown to reduce and/or cure migraines in some people. For those the diet helps, the behavior changes can be modified over time, followed less strictly, perhaps because the brain chemistry has changed as a result of the body's time in ketosis.

The benefits of a ketogenic diet have been seen in those with epilepsy as well. After two years, 50 percent of epilepsy patients who discontinue the diet continue to have the same benefits/seizure reduction they experienced while on the diet. That sounds curative to me. For some, it is.

Interestingly, research as far back as 1928 has shown the ketogenic diet to be effective for migraines. For some reason, this finding wasn't compelling enough, because the next scientific publication didn't surface for another 78 years. Several case reports came out in the early 2000s pointing to the ketogenic diet as helpful for migraines.

Over the past several years, studies have continued to show that the ketogenic diet is effective for treating migraines. According to research done by Dr. Cherubino Di Lorenzo at Sapienza University of Rome and his colleagues, once patients resumed a "normal" high-carbohydrate diet, their headaches began to worsen again.

Maybe you've tried several things and you're wondering why this book will be different. Let me tell you why: Over the past few years, people have finally accepted that a ketogenic diet can be great for treating neurological conditions. Since the diet is much more popular in mainstream culture, many new recipes and keto products have been developed. People no longer think you are crazy if you restrict sugar and eat healthy foods. Many restaurants are supporting keto on their menu. Consumers need to evaluate these products and restaurant offerings to ensure they meet the diet standard they are trying to uphold, but this is a great start!

You can expect this book to be practical. Changing how you eat is difficult, to say the least. But if you are ready to commit—I suggest two to three months of a consistent keto lifestyle—you may see drastic changes

in your migraines. You'll find recipes, macro guidelines, weekly plans, and lifestyle advice, all from a realistic point of view.

Can anyone do this? Yes! I believe it's possible for anyone, but you're going to need strong resolve and determination to follow through. For those of you who are ready to commit and begin the journey toward headache freedom, let's get started.

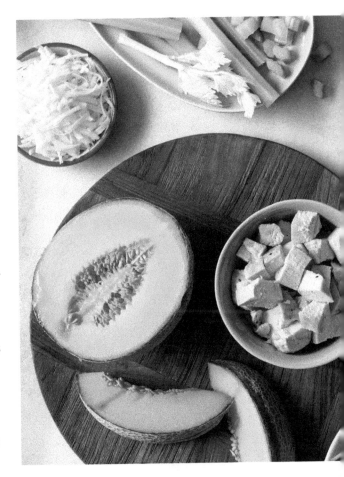

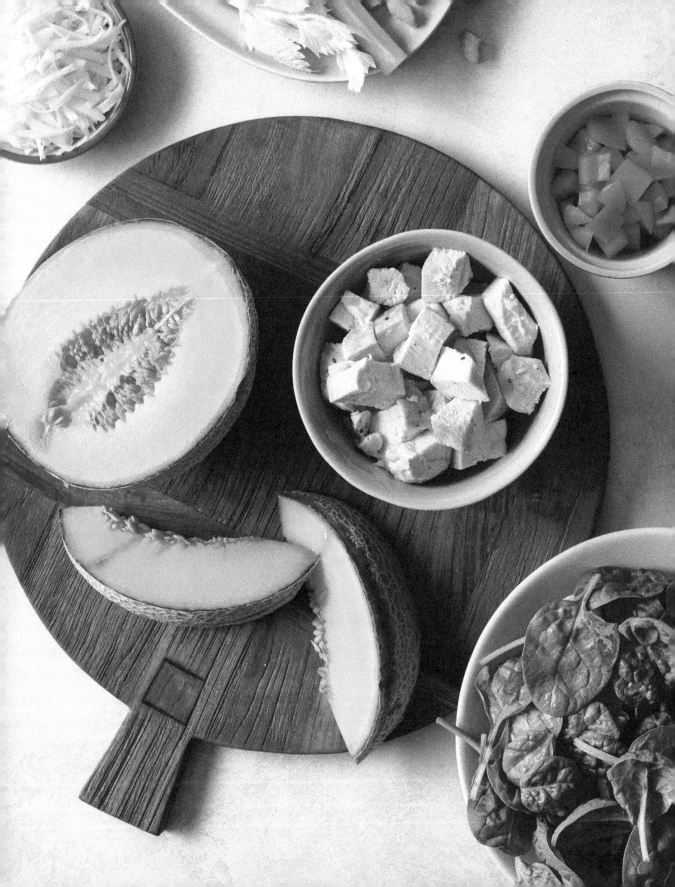

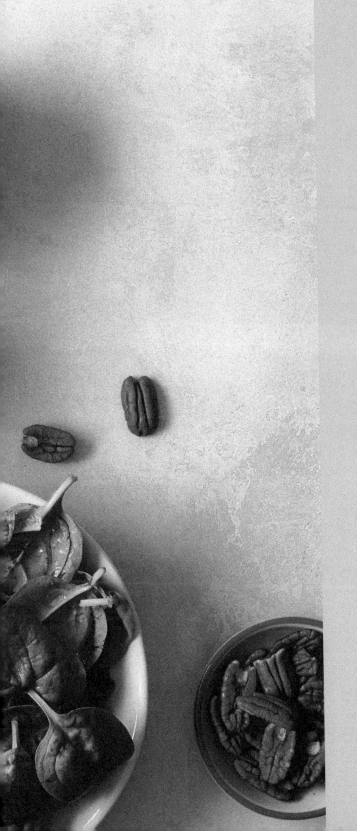

The Healing Power of Food

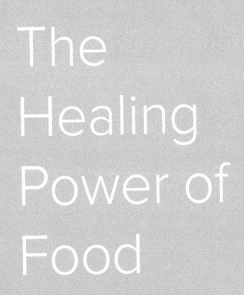

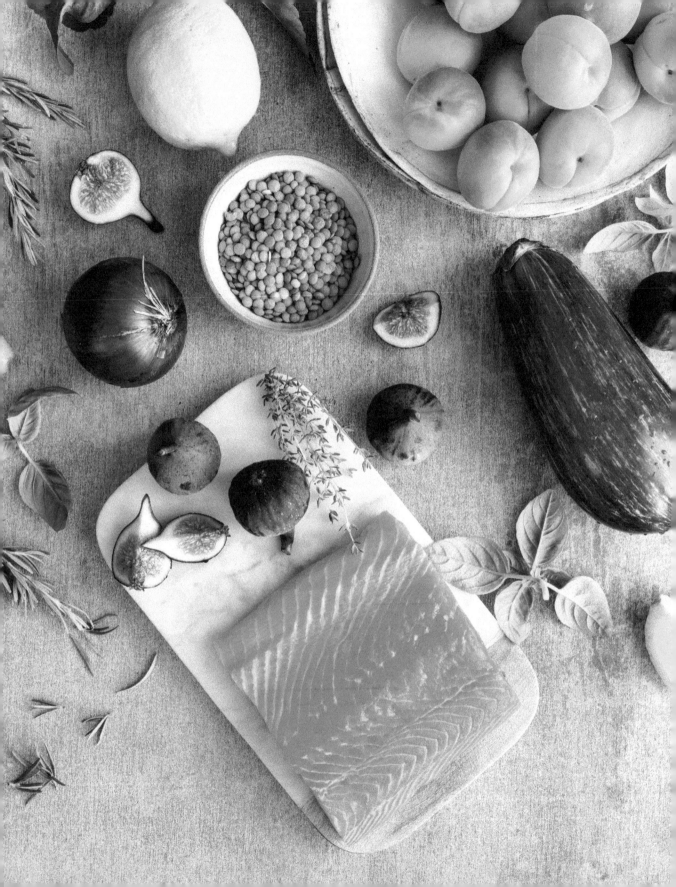

CHAPTER 1

The Problem and the Solution

· ·

Since you're reading this, it's safe to assume that you or a loved one is suffering from migraine headaches. Please prepare yourself to be educated, challenged, and stretched. It's time to learn about a better way to treat migraines—one that your doctor may not have mentioned. It's time for a solution that may finally work.

More Than a Headache

Migraines mean something different to everyone. What exactly is a migraine headache? Here's a technical definition from Harvard Health:

The migraine headache, with or without aura . . . produces pain that usually begins . . . on one side of the head. A migraine headache also often has a pulsating quality to it. Many people experience nausea, extreme sensitivity to light or sound, or both.

If you're close to anyone who suffers from migraines, they may have expressed frustration over missing days of work and pleasure. You may have heard stories of hiding in a darkened room for a day, or many days, hoping the incessant pain would diminish. They may have lost their job, left college, or abandoned their hobbies because of the debilitating effects of these persistent headaches. You may wonder why doctors and current medications can't help them—no one seems to know.

This book's main goal is to offer migraine sufferers hope through a plan based on the latest medical research. This approach is a change for most people and quite a radical transformation for some. But keep in mind that many people have found that a ketogenic diet has improved or even cured their migraine headaches. It's time to join them.

A Way Out

Most of you have surely tried various over-the-counter or prescription medications, with no appreciable benefit. Despite how much knowledge exists about the pathophysiology of migraines, commonly available preventive treatments are effective in only about half of patients.

Introducing . . . the ketogenic diet: a high-fat, low-carbohydrate, moderate-protein eating plan.

BRAIN FOOD

The ketogenic diet has been used as a medical treatment for epilepsy since 1921, when it was discovered that fasting improved and even cured epilepsy. Some patients fasted for up to 21 days. During these fasts, researchers discovered that the patient's body was breaking down fat, which produced ketone bodies. These ketone bodies then become an alternative source of energy for the body. Scientists figured out that by feeding the body a very high percentage of fat, it could be tricked into a state similar to fasting. Even though patients were eating adequate calories, their bodies were induced into this physical state, called ketosis. Ketosis is a metabolic process during which the body burns fat, rather than carbohydrates, for energy.

We've also started to see other medical conditions improve from a keto diet. Conditions such as Alzheimer's disease, Parkinson's disease, and ALS have shown a decrease in symptoms. Some cancers have slowed, stopped growing, or gone into remission per case reports and mounting clinical evidence, especially in glioblastomas. Autistic patients are learning at an increasing rate, and, of course, migraine headaches are resolving.

Why does the keto diet work in people with migraines? One thought is that the state of induced ketosis may favorably restore brain metabolism and excitability and reduce neuro-inflammation. Another idea is that several interacting mechanisms may be at work in the clinical and neurophysiological actions stimulated by a keto diet.

To be honest, researchers don't know the exact mechanisms behind many of the medications we use—they only know that they work. It's the same for the ketogenic diet. There is science to show that it frequently provides relief from migraines, but we don't know exactly why yet.

CUT SIMPLE CARBS

What's so wrong with carbohydrates that we need to eliminate many of them to help fight migraines?

Carbohydrates are compounds made up of sugars, starches, and cellulose, which is fiber. They are easily broken down by the body during digestion, and the body uses them to make glucose.

Simple carbohydrates, which are the most readily digested, are found in fruits, dairy, and some vegetables. Complex carbohydrates take more effort to break down and are found in legumes, most vegetables, whole-grain breads, and cereals.

Because they are digested quickly, simple carbs cause a rapid rise in glucose (blood sugar). Although we don't know why a keto diet, or being in ketosis, improves migraines, we do know that spikes in glucose eliminate ketosis—it's that simple. It's nearly impossible to maintain a state of ketosis while ingesting a significant level of simple carbs (or too many complex carbs, for that matter).

I love fruit as much as the next person, and in general, it's not a bad thing. But many therapeutic diets eliminate certain healthy foods to help treat the medical condition a patient is trying to solve. Take bananas, for example. They are an excellent source of potassium and fiber, but one medium banana provides up to 27 grams of carbohydrates. That amount may be all the carbs you should have in a whole day while using the keto diet to fight migraines.

If bananas are off the table, what do you do for potassium? Try an avocado, the ultimate keto food! One avocado has double the potassium and four times the fiber of a banana. It also provides substantial fat, which is essential for great ketosis.

GET NUTRIENT-DENSE

Much of the food in a typical American diet provides very few nutrients. Take something like wheat bread, for example. Most of the micronutrients in wheat are found in the bran, which is removed during processing. To get the bread back up to a similar level of nutrients, and add a few more, it's enriched with iron, thiamin (B1), niacin (B2), and folic acid. Some breads are even enriched with calcium, a process that was, understandably, started to minimize nutritional deficiencies in whole populations. Ideally, though, we should work to get our nutrients from whole, unprocessed foods as much as possible.

The most nutrient-dense vegetables and fruits are the ones that have the most color: Green, red, orange, and yellow produce is a great source of micronutrients, phytochemicals, fiber, and often prebiotics (food for probiotics). On a keto diet, you get more bang for your buck when vegetables are your main carb source. You can eat a small amount of fruit, but it's harder to incorporate the necessary fats into a meal if your only source of carbohydrates is fruit. Vegetables such as spinach, kale, bell peppers, carrots, broccoli, and asparagus are great, and the few fruits that we'll gravitate toward in this book are avocados (yes, they're a fruit!), strawberries, raspberries, and blackberries.

Protein is another important part of the keto diet. You may need to limit processed foods, such as hot dogs, sausage, and bacon, but overall, it's great to get your protein from several sources. Beef, chicken, pork, fish, lamb, shellfish, eggs, and cheese can all be included, as long as you have no allergies and don't identify these as foods that trigger your migraines. When considering trigger foods, keep in mind that quantity may matter. The amount of protein on a true, therapeutic ketogenic diet is limited to your recommended dietary allowance, so you may find yourself consuming less protein than before.

Behind the Pain

Researchers are working to identify the exact cause of migraines, and, understandably, it's a multifaceted process. We do know that migraines have a genetic component. They are more likely to run in families, and when an identical twin has migraines, the other twin's chance of suffering from them is doubled. We also know that women are three times more likely to have migraines than men.

Let's break this down into the types of migraine headaches and the typical four stages of an attack.

MIGRAINES WITH AURA

About 20 percent of migraine sufferers will have an aura precipitating the actual headache. Auras present in a variety of ways. The most common are flashes of bright light, foggy vision, zigzag lines, small, bright dots, blank spots in vision, and/or feeling like you are looking through heat waves or water.

In my case, once an aura started, I might as well head for home. It was difficult to read due to the blank spots in my vision, not to mention the squiggly flashing lines that were constantly before my eyes. The actual headache would likely start within the next hour, and, interestingly, the aura completely stopped before the headache started. For a moment, I would think I was home free, but more than likely the headache was coming next. If it's truly a migraine, it will probably last at least four hours and as long as three days.

MIGRAINES WITHOUT AURA

A migraine without aura offers little or no warning that a crushing headache is about to begin. The pain of a migraine varies among individuals, but there are common features. A migraine often pulsates, and the pain may be on one side of the head. The pain is generally moderate to severe, which is why it can be difficult for someone to continue with daily activities. Many people are very sensitive to sound and light and find they must retreat to an extremely quiet, darkened room.

Other less common classifications of migraines exist, and some people can have a migraine that doesn't involve pain at all. Instead, they may have visual disturbances, dizziness, and speech issues, but it never evolves into pain.

A MIGRAINE'S PATH

Migraines often present in four stages:

Prodrome: Begins a few hours to a few days before the migraine; experienced by one-third of sufferers. Common symptoms: irritability; depression; yawning; increased urination; food cravings; light/sound sensitivity; difficulty concentrating; fatigue and muscle stiffness; difficulty speaking, reading, and sleeping; nausea.

Aura: Begins 5 to 60 minutes before the headache; experienced by one-fifth of people suffering from migraines. Common symptoms: visual disturbances (flashes of light, blind spots in vision), temporary loss of vision, numbness, tingling.

Attack/Headache: May last 4 to 72 hours; experienced by most migraine sufferers. Common symptoms: throbbing pain in the head (drilling, icepick, burning); nausea; vomiting; giddiness; insomnia; congestion; anxiety; depressed mood; sensitivity to light, smell, and sound; neck pain; stiffness.

Postdrome/Hangover: May last 24 to 48 hours; experienced by three-fourths of people with migraines. Common symptoms: inability to concentrate, fatigue, depressed mood, euphoric mood, lack of comprehension, nausea.

A MEDICAL MYSTERY

Even with years of research into the reasons behind migraines, scientists are still working to determine their actual cause, the mechanisms involved, and how to best prevent them. It's understood that there is a genetic component as well as an altered brain biology. It's also known that many migraines arise from some sort of trigger. Genetic testing is beginning to unlock some of this knowledge, but such findings may turn into even more unanswered questions. Brain processes are complex, and for now, many of the answers about how migraines arise continue to puzzle researchers.

Common Medical Interventions

Many of you are probably familiar with the common interventions for migraines, but let's review the most traditional methods.

PAIN RELIEVERS

Ergot: Dihydroergotamine and ergotamine are medications used to treat severe, throbbing headaches. They have a severe side-effect profile and interact with numerous other drugs. They are useful only for headache pain.

Opioids: These addictive painkillers (Oxycontin, Vicodin, Percocet) are prescribed for 50 percent of migraine emergency room visits. According to Dr. Stephen Silberstein, director of the Headache Center at Jefferson University Hospital, opioids may be necessary in certain situations, but otherwise may lead to addiction and could even cause frequent migraines to evolve into chronic migraines.

NSAIDs: Nonsteroidal anti-inflammatory drugs (Ibuprofen, Naproxen), if selected and prescribed wisely, are safe and cost-effective for treating migraine attacks.

PREVENTIVE

For preventive therapy, numerous medications may be considered: beta-blockers, anti-convulsants, anti-depressants, calcium-channel blockers, angiotensin blockers, NSAIDs, triptans, and calcitonin gene-related peptide therapy. Each of these has a different level of effectiveness, with beta-blockers and anti-convulsants leading the way with the best results. A two- to three-month trial of each medication is needed to fully assess efficacy, and it may take up to six months to fully evaluate the treatment. Each of these medications comes with its own side-effect profile, some worse than others.

Topiramate is an anti-convulsant that is commonly used for migraine prevention. One study found that topiramate reduced headaches by one day per month—the same effect as adding 40 minutes of exercise per week.

BOTOX

Botox injections for chronic migraines (more than 15 episodes per month) have shown to be only modestly effective. In a 2012 paper in the *Journal of the American Medical Association* that reviewed data from 27 trials, Botox was found to reduce chronic migraine headaches by two migraines per month.

TRANSCRANIAL MAGNETIC STIMULATION (TMS)

A TMS device has been FDA-approved since 2013 and is occasionally used for patients who are unable to take medications for their condition. The device is handheld and uses magnets to stimulate the brain once a migraine has started. It can be used once per day and has shown to be somewhat more effective than not treating the migraine at all.

GOODBYE, GLUTEN?

Some people identify gluten as a migraine trigger. The ketogenic diet is nearly gluten-free due to the limited carbohydrates. If you perceive gluten to be a trigger for you, by all means avoid it. Most of the recipes in this book are gluten-free—and the few that aren't can easily be modified.

Supplemental Therapies

Many migraine sufferers prefer to treat or prevent their headaches without medications. Every medication has potential side effects and they don't work for everyone. Interestingly enough, many nonmedication therapies have a similar effectiveness to commonly prescribed medications. Some migraine sufferers use medications along with other therapies they find to be helpful.

ACUPUNCTURE

Acupuncture can be helpful for many things beyond pain control. It's also used to maintain good health and address the body's life energy, or *qi*. The goal of great acupuncture is to restore the balance between one's body, spirit, and emotions.

There is quite a debate in the medical community regarding acupuncture and its usefulness for migraine prevention. Thankfully, this has been fairly well-studied with confirmed positive results. According to Dr. Kien Trinh of McMaster University in Ontario and his colleagues, moderate evidence suggests that for episodic migraine prevention, acupuncture is "at least noninferior" to now-proven conventional treatments.

MASSAGE THERAPY

Since stress is such an identifiable trigger for migraines, it would be logical to consider that massage may have a place in migraine prevention and treatment. A study in the *International Journal of Neuroscience* showed a reduction in several migraine-related variables after 10 weeks of twice-weekly massages. Patients had a statistically significant decrease in intensity, frequency, and duration of their migraines. Massage may be a nice addition to someone's overall program; if nothing else, it feels great and is relaxing.

COGNITIVE THERAPIES

Of the 76 percent of people who report occasionally having migraine triggers, 8 out of 10 cite stress as their number one trigger. It makes sense that reducing and managing stress would be beneficial for those suffering from migraines. Cognitive behavioral therapy (CBT) is led by a psychologist who uses relaxation and coping strategies, assertive communication, and stress management to help people decrease the frequency, intensity, and duration of migraine headaches. According to the Association of Migraine Disorders, existing literature shows that CBT decreases headache activity by 30 to 60 percent. That's nearly as good as medication, and it offers positive side effects, not harmful ones like many medications do.

THE MIGRAINE DIARY

To determine your migraine triggers, keep a headache diary. This template will help you identify patterns that coincide with your attacks.

Date and day of the week ....

What time did the migraine start?

....

How long did the migraine last?

....

Did you do anything to treat it? Did it work?

....

What were you doing leading up to the attack?

....

How many hours did you sleep the previous night?

....

What did you eat in the 24 hours before the attack?

....

What medications were you taking at the time?

....

Have you recently experienced any major life changes or stresses?

....

Please remember that you should always consult your physician for treatment strategies. This book is not meant to replace your primary medical doctor.

Freedom from Migraines

We've covered a lot of information. We've discussed many aspects of your life and your health and considered numerous ways to improve both. Now let's move forward and begin putting legs on these goals. Good intentions are just that—intentions. Action is now required.

FIVE STEPS TO FREEDOM

In the chapters that follow, you will learn how to take the outlined plan and incorporate it into your life. In the next chapter, we will embark on a process, Five Steps to Freedom, that will prepare you for the lifestyle changes necessary to achieve the greatest success. Each section is critical in its own way. Take your time as you read each step. Think about these steps, meditate on them, and discuss them with your family or support system.

MEAL PLAN

This is what you've been waiting for: how to design your day's meals with the best configuration for your macronutrients, or macros. Macros (carbs, protein, and fat) are the main source of your calories (carbs, protein, and fat) and must be distributed properly within the ketogenic diet to obtain the best ketosis and the best chance of migraine relief.

The meal plan should be relatively easy to follow, once you understand some of the basic concepts behind the ketogenic diet. It won't come naturally to many people, as the keto way of eating can be a bit counterintuitive. Many of us, for example, have been raised and trained to think of fat as evil. But it's not evil—it's an important contributor to the keto diet. (You'll find some sample macros in the box on page 13, and I'll explain more about the keto ratio on page 26.)

CALCULATING YOUR MACROS

Everyone has different calorie needs. You can get a rough idea of your estimated caloric needs by using one of the recommended apps listed in the Resources on page 213. In general, though, try to keep the percentage of fat in your daily diet at 70 to 80 percent, carbohydrates at 5 to 10 percent, and protein at 12 to 20 percent. This will put your ketogenic ratio in the 1:1 to 2:1 range.

Here are some macro estimates for daily consumption of 1,500 and 2,000 calories.

> 1,500 calories: 115g fat, 30g carbs, 85g protein (1:1 keto ratio)
> 1,500 calories: 128g fat, 20g carbs, 66g protein (1.5:1 keto ratio)
> 1,500 calories: 136g fat, 13g carbs, 55g protein (2:1 keto ratio)
> 2,000 calories: 154g fat, 35g carbs, 119g protein (1:1 keto ratio)
> 2,000 calories: 170g fat, 25g carbs, 90g protein (1.5:1 keto ratio)
> 2,000 calories: 180g fat, 25g carbs, 66g protein (2:1 keto ratio)

I recommend you track all of your foods during the first month on the plan. These numbers may be adjusted to your particular situation. If your goal is to lose weight, keep in mind that the truth will be told by whether you lose, gain, or maintain your weight at a certain calorie level. Adjust your calories as needed to meet weight goals.

Please note that the recommended daily allowance for protein for adults is 0.8g per kg of body weight. This may be adjusted downward if you are significantly overweight. You can also move protein up and carbs down, or vice versa, within the guidelines above to best meet your needs and situation.

RECIPES

The recipes in this book include everything from appetizers to snacks, from simple breakfast smoothies to lovely dinners. They have been designed with a busy person in mind. Most of us need to find something to prepare that is relatively simple, quick, and tasty. Our patience is thin when it comes to meals that aren't flavorful.

And desserts—let's not forget desserts! You will be pleasantly surprised at the variety of sweet offerings. It's okay to have some sweets, as long as they're keto-approved. You'll see that as long as you don't find stevia or erythritol to be a trigger, desserts can usually be incorporated into your diet in small amounts. Please avoid them if you have any concerns.

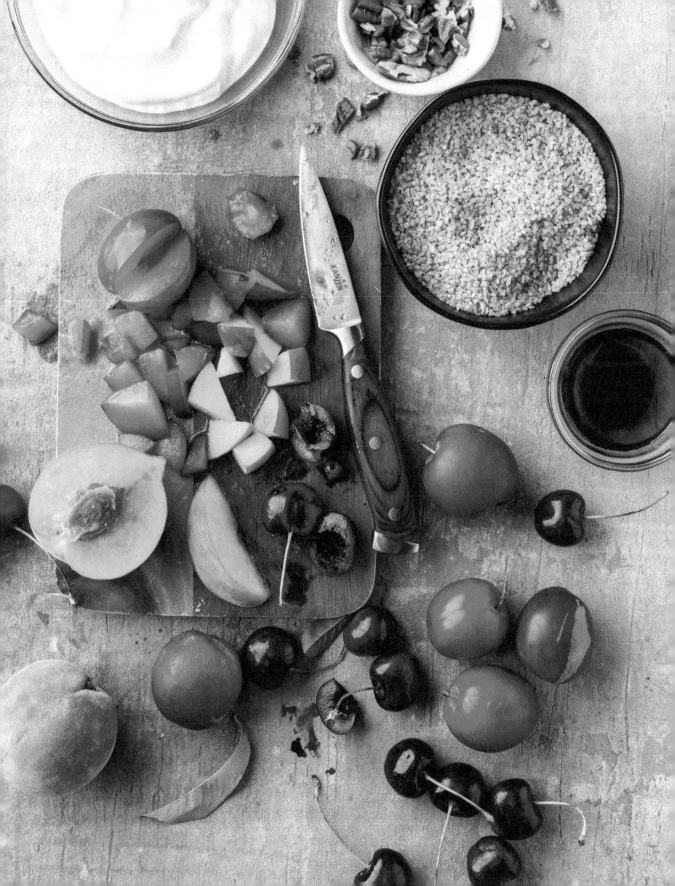

CHAPTER 2

The Foundations

. . . .

Now let's get down to the meat and potatoes (or should I say, meat and cauliflower rice) of this plan. We will gently walk through five steps that will lead you to a successful ketogenic strategy to fight migraines.

How do you learn to walk? One step at a time. Please don't try to start out running on this plan—it's easy to trip and fall if you're not prepared. And if you fall, it can be difficult to get back up. Make sure to read through each section before you begin.

Step 1: Commit

We commit to things that are noble, good, and healthy all the time. We purchase a gym membership with plans to work out three times a week. We volunteer at our favorite organization because we believe in the cause. But sometimes, after a few weeks or months, we grow tired of the commitment and we bail.

This is going to take effort. This program isn't worth doing if you're not willing to put a tremendous amount of time and attention into your health.

I challenge you to put most of your efforts into Step 1 before you move forward with any further steps. There is no guaranteed length of time within which you will see results with your migraines. While I know people who have seen results in only a few days, I urge you to commit a full three months to this program. That seems like a long time, but is it as much as all the time you've lost to migraines?

Keep in mind that when this diet is used to treat epilepsy, a three-month trial is recommended. It can take that long for the chemical changes in the brain to have full impact. We aren't dealing with epilepsy here, but we are dealing with a very complex brain. We have to give it time.

Step 2: Pantry Clean-Out

Once you have committed to changing your diet, you will probably see the advantage in preparing your kitchen. There are foods that may be technically healthy that you will need to avoid or limit in order to achieve and maintain ketosis. I realize that restricting entire food groups like grains and fruits is extreme. I'm not suggesting that everyone needs to restrict carbohydrates to a medically therapeutic level, just as a doctor would never suggest that someone without migraines take a daily medication to prevent them.

As you move forward with the pantry clean-out, remember that you are doing yourself a favor in the long run. The favor may be a migraine-free life!

PARE DOWN YOUR PANTRY

If you live alone, this will be fairly easy. If you have a spouse, a roommate, or a family, you should probably have a chat with them first. You might be pleasantly surprised at what those around you are willing to do—after all, they want you to feel better. It might take some effort on their end to make this work for you, but don't be afraid to tell them that their help and cooperation are essential to your success.

TOSS LIST

Cereal, bread, granola bars (even the "healthy" ones), rice, pasta, crackers, croutons, white sugar, brown sugar, powdered sugar, flour, white and sweet potatoes, gluten-free products that contain significant carbohydrate amounts, sweets (cookies, snack cakes, ice cream, cake, pie, candy), soup, processed boxed mixes, chips, ketchup, barbecue sauce, margarine, sweet salad dressing, sweet pickles, fruit juice, sweet drink mixes, liqueurs, protein powders, and mixes that contain more than 2 grams of carbohydrate per serving

HERE'S WHAT TO KEEP OR STOCK

Oils (especially olive, coconut, avocado, and macadamia), MCT oil (see page 213), mayonnaise, butter, ghee, heavy (whipping) cream, spices and herbs, coconut manna (a kind of butter made from ground coconut with the water removed), cocoa powder, vinegars, fresh and frozen vegetables, berries, fruit (eaten minimally, but okay on occasion), beef, pork, lamb, chicken, seafood, eggs, hard cheeses, nuts (macadamia, pecans, walnuts, and pili nuts are best), nut butters, almond flour, coconut flour, chia seeds, ground flax, unsweetened full-fat yogurt, unsweetened kefir, fermented vegetables, avocados, olives, coconut cream, coconut milk, unsweetened almond milk, cream cheese, sour cream, hemp hearts, sweeteners (erythritol, stevia, and monk fruit)

It's great to eat organic fruits and vegetables, grass-fed proteins, and minimally processed foods as much as your budget allows.

VITAMINS AND SUPPLEMENTS

There are many opinions about whether nutritional supplementation has a place in migraine treatment and prevention. Some studies show a benefit, while others do not. Individuals may find that their benefit is worthwhile, with a significant reduction in headaches.

Here are some to consider.

Multivitamin: While following a ketogenic diet, a multivitamin supplement with iron is recommended due to the restrictive nature of the diet. In order to decrease carbohydrates enough to promote ketosis, nutrients are often sacrificed.

Calcium: Calcium is a recommended supplement for keto diets. Dairy products are quite limited on the keto diet because it avoids milk and limits yogurt (which contain natural sugar/carbs). Cheese has great calcium levels, but you would need three to four ounces per day to provide enough calcium. Consider taking 50 to 100 percent of your Dietary Reference Intake (DRI) for calcium daily from a respected supplement. The DRI for most adults ranges from 800mg to 1,000mg per day.

Vitamin D: This is often taken in moderate doses along with a keto diet, because of the drastic dietary changes required and the potential for insufficiency. My experience has been that people tend to need many times the DRI in order to keep their levels in the normal range. In the case of low blood levels of vitamin D in conjunction with migraine headaches, it is definitely beneficial to supplement vitamin D to bring the blood within normal ranges, which improves headaches.

Potassium: Intake of this nutrient is frequently low when consuming a ketogenic diet, due to the limitations on certain fruits and vegetables. If you do not have problems with your kidneys, you may benefit from using a salt substitute that contains potassium chloride to season your food and add the needed potassium. Choose a salt substitute that contains potassium chloride combined with sodium chloride (table salt). Please check with your doctor before using a potassium chloride product, and don't use it if you have been told to limit potassium.

Magnesium: Migraine sufferers have been shown to have lower magnesium levels and may benefit from either increased dietary magnesium intake or supplementation. Adequate blood levels will likely help reduce the frequency of headaches. A few good sources of magnesium are avocados, spinach, almonds, cashews, and peanuts.

Coenzyme Q10 (CoQ10): CoQ10 plus nano-curcumin can decrease migraine attacks and their severity. And carnitine, in conjunction with CoQ10, has also shown beneficial effects for migraine symptoms.

Feverfew: There is a 50 percent migraine reduction reported by using a combination of feverfew, CoQ10, riboflavin, and magnesium in children.

Step 3: Get Active

Regular exercise and activity will have great benefits for people with migraines, much as it is a great benefit to everyone. For years, exercise has been shown to reduce the risk of chronic diseases and improve depression, sleep, and mood. If you've ever exercised regularly, you likely have felt the benefits.

Migraines are sometimes the reason that exercise falls by the wayside. For some people, strenuous exercise may induce migraines, so this small subset of people needs to be extra cautious.

MAKE MOVES

Many careers are very sedentary and make it difficult to get a reasonable amount of daily activity. So what can be done? Don't give up. Most people, if they are willing, can start building at least a little activity into their lives. A lot would be great, but a little is at least a start. Exercise has been proven to decrease migraines and even reduce their intensity and duration.

It will be well worth carving out the time to start or increase your physical activity. Think of it like putting together a large puzzle, and exercise is one of the key pieces.

If you feel you absolutely don't have the time to exercise, think again about your weekly schedule and whether there are two or three times a week when you could actually exercise. With a few exceptions, I think everyone can find a few minutes—it comes down to priorities.

ONE STEP AT A TIME

What does exercise mean for you? If you haven't been doing much of it, it might mean going for a nice walk. If you have favorite activities already, it may be something along the lines of jogging, biking, swimming, yoga, or visiting the local gym to use the aerobic machines (treadmill, bikes, Stairmaster, elliptical, and others). There is no one-size-fits-all—it has to fit you. You have to like doing it, or at least not hate it, or you won't stick with it.

30-MINUTE SEQUENCE

To get the most aerobic benefit from exercise, your heart rate needs to go up. A brisk walk is one of the best ways to do this. If you can't find a place to walk, maybe you have access to some type of exercise equipment. Spend 10 to 20 minutes either walking or using the most easily available piece of aerobic equipment. (As always, consult your physician before undertaking any exercise program.)

Remember that your body needs to warm up to reduce your chances of an injury. Please start at whatever is a mild intensity for you for the first few minutes and work your way up. It's also a great idea to do some simple stretches to loosen up your quadriceps, calves, and arms. Please see the Resources section (see page 213) for a great website with pictures of stretches.

Once you've spent 10 to 20 minutes exercising, take a few minutes to wrap it up with a cool-down. Slow your walk to a very casual pace for the last three to five minutes or do the same on the machine of your choice.

For those with limited mobility, a brisk walk or exercise equipment may not be realistic. But there is likely a way to increase your current level of exercise. If you're able to walk but are very limited, perhaps you can do laps around the inside of the house. Or you could sit in your favorite chair and use cans of soup as weights and get some arm exercise. Maybe watch a YouTube video on chair yoga (and do it, don't just watch!).

With few exceptions, we can all do something to increase our fitness level and contribute toward overall healing of our body and migraines.

Step 4: Align Your Body with Your Mind

When our physical bodies begin to suffer, our minds can quickly follow. Just as we have to train our physical bodies, we must also train our minds. This may be even more important than your physical activity. If your mind is out of alignment, every other area of your life will suffer.

PSYCHOLOGICAL WELLNESS

At the beginning of a migraine, are you stressed, upset, discouraged? Does the mere fact that a headache is looming cause your mind to go in a dozen different directions? This is an emotional hit for most people, but the frustration and tension don't have to make your migraine worse—not if you have a plan.

Cognitive behavioral therapy (CBT) involves many different components, but no one truly masters all of them. Each person would be well-served to look at their own situation and determine what aspect of CBT would be the most beneficial to them. Three areas to think about first would be mindfulness, meditation, and stress reduction.

MINDFULNESS, MEDITATION, AND STRESS REDUCTION

Mindfulness is defined as the self-regulation of attention with an attitude of curiosity, openness, and acceptance. But what does that mean in real life? It means to be present in the here and now, to narrow your attention, regulate your focus, and learn during the process.

Learning to control negative thoughts and subsequent actions will begin to decrease your stress level and may aid in reducing migraines and lessen the severity of the attacks.

Meditation is practiced in many ways. Some may pray and meditate, while others may just relax, focus, and clear their minds. And there are those who may focus on an object, issue, or activity in order to bring clarity. In a culture where we are too busy to relax, where our days are packed and time seems to run like water through our hands, meditation can be invaluable to those who make time for it.

How many times has someone asked how you are and you responded, "Stressed!" It has become too easy to believe that living in a constant state of stress is normal. It's not normal, nor is it healthy.

Can you identify attitudes, people, or places that aren't healthy for you and that cause undue stress? Take a moment to consider your life. Evaluate what is going on, in, and around you and decide what needs to change. Can you keep living with your current level of stress?

MEDITATION: EXPLORING PAIN

"You are what you are and where you are because of what has gone into your mind. You can change what you are and where you are by changing what goes into your mind."

—Zig Ziglar

Meditation is often overlooked when it comes to our health. Garbage put into our mind translates into just that—garbage in our mind. You can't avoid bad thoughts—they happen. Sometimes they build up and sometimes we feed them and help them to grow into terrible thoughts. How do you stop this cycle and how does it relate to your migraines?

Learning to focus your thoughts and relax your mind takes discipline. Find a quiet spot, sit, relax, and just breathe for a minute. During that time, think only about your breath, nothing else. You may find that you can't even go a full minute without a rush of ideas, plans, and commitments jumping into your brain. Don't be surprised—you're not alone.

You may find that learning to meditate helps you gain focus, better manage your pain, and lowers your stress. (There are places to find more tips and advice listed in the Resources section on page 213.)

Step 5: Get Prepared

Most often, we succeed in a new venture because we have prepared to such a level that success naturally follows. Don't expect this journey will be any different. Your hard work, attention to details, and commitment will be responsible for your success.

ESTABLISH A ROUTINE

Creating a structure for your shopping and food preparation will be invaluable as you begin this process. Diet modifications can be difficult, so creating a framework before you start is essential. Consider how often you need to shop (at least weekly). How often will you cook and do food prep? Are you willing to eat leftovers or do you prefer fresh meals every day?

Please consider putting your routine in writing; you will likely find that words on paper are motivating and promote the importance of the task at hand.

MAKE THE TIME

The recipes and ideas in this book are designed with you in mind. I assume you have a busy life and have certain times that you don't feel well because of migraines. To be successful on this plan, you must carve out the time to shop and cook. Sure, you can eat out on occasion, but you'll do better when you can be in complete control of what goes into and on your food.

Take a few minutes each week to pick out meals and recipes for the upcoming week. Choose them far enough in advance that you have time to shop for ingredients. It will be very satisfying to know what you plan to cook and eat on any given day.

FORGIVE FUMBLES

Let's establish right now that you won't do this perfectly. There may be a day when you give in to a craving, skip your exercise, forget to shop, or have no time to cook. Expect this—it's life.

Possibly the most important piece of your plan, yet one that's often forgotten, is accountability. A program started without accountability is more easily abandoned than one that you have told others about.

True accountability is most useful when there is a person or a group that is specifically checking in and encouraging you. This may be a spouse, a friend, or a medical professional such as a Registered Dietitian Nutritionist. Choose your accountability partner or group carefully. It should be someone who really will check in with you and ask you the hard questions.

FIND THE FUN

If you are dreading the start of a new way of eating, please step back a moment. Attitude is at least 90 percent of life, so consider that this may be the beginning of something beautiful. Do you like to try new recipes? Great. If not, is there someone in your family who does and may be interested in helping?

Have you ever found the time to exercise or meditate? Getting ahold of your life and your health has so many rewards. You will likely enjoy reaping the benefits of the changes you've made. And as you begin to feel better, you will find more and more activities to do that you've been missing because of the headaches.

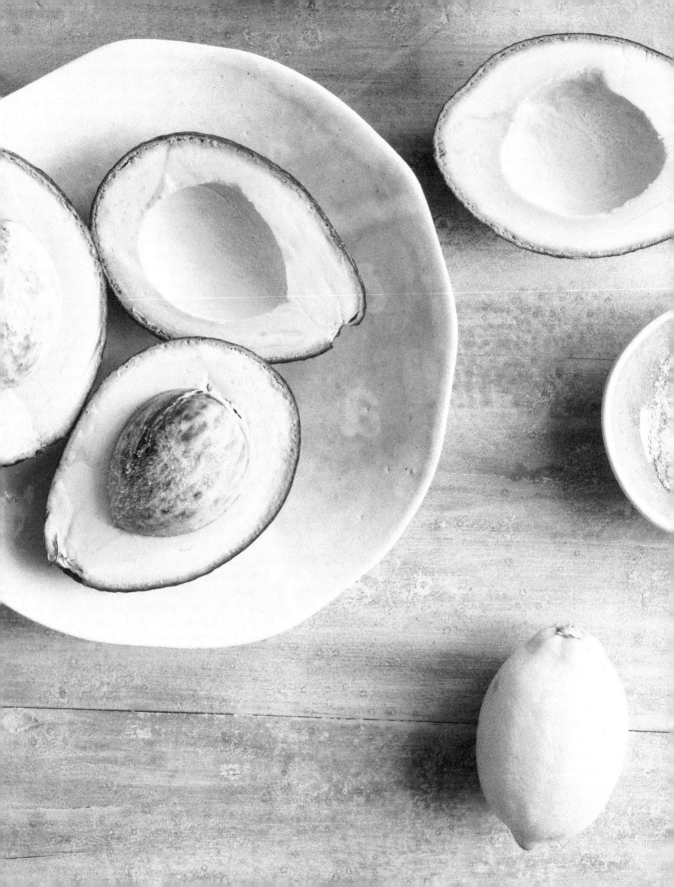

CHAPTER 3

The Plan

. . . .

We've reached the crux of this book: the delicious recipes and meal plans that will propel you into successful ketogenic therapy. You will notice that Week One is a slow, nonspecific transition into the plan. There is a great reason for this: If you start out with a very low-carb diet too quickly, you may become acidotic (also known as the keto flu; see page 32) and feel miserable. A gentle transition will help you avoid this entirely.

As we move into Week Two, you'll see I've included options for something quick so you can grab and go, as well as lovely meals that you will be proud to serve to your friends and family.

I've sketched out four weeks, 21 days of meal plans here, but of course you can adjust these to meet your lifestyle and needs. Many of these meals can be completed in 30 minutes or less. So stick with the plan, remember your "why," and let's keep this going for the full four weeks.

You may need to extend the diet up to three months to see the full benefit of the ketogenic diet. If you see results, it will be best to continue the meal plan. No one knows how long the diet must be followed—the answer is likely different for everyone.

THE KETO RATIO

The ratio of fat to net carbohydrates plus protein in a food is known as the keto-genic ratio. To keep your body in ketosis, you need to maintain the right ratio throughout the day. I recommend a ratio of 1:1 to 2:1 at each meal for most adults.

The first number in the ratio is grams of fat, and the second number is grams of protein plus grams of net carbohydrates (that's grams of total carbs minus grams of fiber). For example:

1 ounce of almonds has 16g of fat, 6g of protein, and 2g of net carbohydrates (5g of total carbohydrates minus 3g of fiber)

> Ketogenic ratio = 16g fat:6g protein + 2g net carbs
> 16:8 (added 6 + 2)
> 2:1 (reduced the fraction)

You will find the ketogenic ratios for one serving of each recipe in this book in the nutritional information at the end of the recipe.

Refresh and Restock

We've already discussed in chapter 1 what to remove from your kitchen and what's okay to keep. Now let's look at some of the specifics you need to add so you have all the right ingredients. These lists represent all of the ingredients used in the recipes. Rely on the weekly shopping list for what to buy each week.

THE BASICS (STAPLES)

- Almond flour
- Almond meal
- Apple cider vinegar
- Avocado oil
- Avocado oil mayonnaise
- Balsamic vinaigrette
- Beef stock (low-sodium)

- Cacao powder or unsweetened cocoa powder
- Chicken stock (low-sodium)
- Cocoa butter (or cacao butter)
- Coconut flour
- Coconut milk (canned), full-fat
- Coconut oil

- Curry paste
- Fish sauce
- Konjac noodles
- Olive oil
- Olive oil spray
- Protein powder, vanilla (no sugar-added) (small can)
- Pure vanilla extract
- Sesame oil
- Soy sauce (MSG-free)
- Sriracha hot sauce
- Swerve sweetener (or an erythritol-stevia blend sweetener)
- Thai red curry paste
- Tofu, firm
- Tomato paste (low-sodium)
- Tomato sauce (low-sodium and sugar-free)
- Vegetable stock (low-sodium)

HERBS AND SPICES

- Ancho chili powder
- Basil (fresh)
- Bay leaves (fresh or dried)
- Black pepper
- Cayenne pepper
- Chipotle chili powder
- Chives (fresh)
- Cilantro (fresh)
- Cinnamon (ground)
- Cloves (ground)
- Coriander (ground)
- Cumin (ground)
- Fennel seed
- Garlic (fresh)
- Garam masala
- Ginger (fresh)
- Mint (fresh)
- Nutmeg (ground)
- Paprika
- Parsley (fresh)
- Red pepper flakes
- Sea salt
- Thyme (fresh)
- Turmeric (ground)

FRUITS AND VEGETABLES

Including healthy vegetables and fruits in the plan is essential to ensure maximum nutrition, prebiotics, and fiber. The meal plans offer a variety of nutrients that are all essential to your overall health. Purchase fresh produce whenever possible, but frozen and canned are also acceptable.

- Asparagus
- Avocado
- Bean sprouts
- Bell peppers (red, yellow, and green)
- Blackberries
- Blueberries
- Bok choy
- Broccoli
- Brussels sprouts
- Cabbage
- Cantaloupe
- Cauliflower
- Celery
- Cucumber
- Eggplant
- English cucumber
- Fennel
- Jalapeño pepper

- Jicama
- Kale
- Leek
- Lemon
- Lime
- Mixed greens
- Napa cabbage
- Okra
- Olives (black and Kalamata)
- Pumpkin (raw or frozen)
- Radish
- Raspberries (fresh or frozen)
- Scallions
- Spaghetti squash
- Spinach (fresh)
- Strawberries
- Sweet onion
- Swiss chard
- Watercress
- Zucchini (green and yellow)

ANIMAL PROTEINS

This plan is generally aimed at omnivores (those who eat vegetables and meat), but see the Meatless Mains chapter (see page 123) for a nice selection of vegetarian meals. It's fine to eat different types of protein on a keto diet, even if they are low-fat. You can easily increase the fat in other areas of the meal.

- Bacon (uncured)
- Beef chuck roast
- Chicken breast
- Crab
- Eggs
- Flank steak
- Ground beef
- Ground lamb
- Ground turkey
- Haddock
- Lamb chops
- Lamb racks
- Mussels
- Pork belly
- Pork rib chop
- Rib eye steak
- Salmon (wild-caught)
- Scallops
- Shrimp
- Sole
- Tilapia
- Tuna
- Trout
- Turkey
- Whole roasting chicken

NUTS AND SEEDS

Nuts and seeds are naturally high in fat and make great choices for a healthy keto diet. They contain a few carbohydrates, but this is fine in the nutritional big picture.

- Almond butter (natural)
- Brazil nuts
- Chia seeds
- Coconut, shredded (unsweetened)
- Macadamia nuts
- Peanut butter (natural)
- Peanuts
- Pecans
- Pumpkin seeds
- Sesame seeds

DAIRY

Dairy may be consumed on a ketogenic diet if you have no allergies or intolerances. You should avoid it, of course, if it is a migraine trigger for you. Keep in mind that any trigger may depend on how much of an item you eat. You may tolerate small amounts with no consequences. Substitutions can be made in most recipes.

Please use only full-fat dairy products. Do not choose low-fat, lite, or fat-free dairy products, as these will not provide adequate fat for ketosis.

- Butter (stick, grass-fed preferred but not required)
- Cheddar cheese
- Cream cheese (blocks, not tubs)
- Gouda cheese
- Heavy (whipping) cream (5 to 6 grams of fat per 15mL serving)
- Jalapeño Cheddar cheese
- Mascarpone cheese
- Mozzarella cheese (fresh)
- Parmesan cheese
- Soft goat cheese
- Sour cream

TRIGGERS AND THRESHOLDS

Many migraine sufferers can usually identify triggers—dietary, emotional, or environmental sources that stimulate a migraine. Triggers can be anything from stress to food to hormones to alcohol. Food may be second only to stress as the most common identifiable trigger. Histamines in foods are often the main culprit and are found in foods such as alcohol (especially red wine and beer), fermented foods, cured meats, aged cheeses, and chocolate. There are small amounts in some vegetables.

Caffeine, whether too much or too little, can also trigger a migraine, as can getting overly hungry. Some people are certain that dairy is problematic for them and others know that gluten is a trigger. Please remember that if gluten is a trigger, you should discuss the possibility of celiac disease with your physician.

Food and stress aren't the only issues. Environmental factors play a part for some people: Bright sunlight, fluorescent lights (especially when flickering), and poor sleep hygiene are all known to be migraine triggers.

There's one last trigger that can be very difficult to control: hormones. Many women have "menstrual migraines" that coincide with their menstrual cycle. These attacks are occasionally helped by birth control methods that alter estrogen levels. Hormones likely explain why migraines are three times as likely to occur in women as in men.

The Functional Kitchen

To cook healthy, appealing meals, you need the right equipment. An ill-equipped kitchen will only frustrate you as you endeavor to make these dietary changes. Perhaps you don't have some of these items yet or are unable to invest in all of them at once. That's fine—take a look at what you have and make a list of the items you need or would just like to have. Perhaps you can purchase these one at a time over the next several weeks or months. Maybe you can ask for a spiralizer for your birthday or the holidays. A great set of knives is imperative and also makes a great gift.

KITCHENWARE

- Baking tray/pan
- Barbecue grill (optional, but adds zest to your meats)
- Blender (great for smoothies)
- Casserole dishes—small, medium, and large
- Cast iron skillet (optional, but enhances some recipes)
- Food processor (to quickly purée soups)
- Ice pop molds (to make fantastic frozen treats)
- Immersion blender (if you don't have a food processor, this cost-effective tool is handy for a quick purée or smoothie)
- Mandolin (to peel, slice, julienne, waffle cut, and more)
- Mixing bowls—small, medium, and large
- Pie pan (for quiches)
- Saucepans—small, medium, and large
- Sieve (filters out unwanted seeds)
- Skillet—large (for cream cheese pancakes and many other dishes)
- Spiralizer (great for making zucchini noodles)
- Springform pan (for beautiful cheesecake)
- Stainless steel bowl—large
- Stockpot (essential for yummy soup recipes)

UTENSILS

You may have most of these items in your kitchen already. Make sure your knives are nice and sharp, so cutting vegetables is a pleasure and not a chore. You may decide to get an inexpensive handheld knife sharpener.

- Aluminum foil
- Chef's knife (great for chopping vegetables)
- Chopper (great for chopping vegetables and saving your fingers from sharp knives)
- Dental floss or fishing line (slices through cheese like magic)
- Large zip-top bags (use for marinades)
- Parchment paper (keeps everything from sticking)
- Paring knife (perhaps the most essential tool in every kitchen)
- Peeler (for peeling but also to shave vegetables to make ribbons)
- Scraper—small and large (don't leave half your smoothie in the blender)
- Slicing/carving knife (fundamental tool for everyday meat slicing)
- Slotted spoon
- Spatula (food must be flipped)
- Whisk (great for mixing eggs or making mayonnaise)
- Wooden spoons (you'll use these to stir everything)

STORAGE SOLUTIONS

For healthy food storage, consider a nice set of glass storage containers in various sizes. They should be safe to use in the freezer, microwave, and oven. Also consider:

- Beeswax wrap (environmentally friendly storage)
- Mason jars (great for storing soups and stews)
- Plastic wrap
- Salad-dressing containers—glass preferred (homemade dressings are excellent)

WEEK ONE

Gradually reducing carbohydrates in your diet will help you avoid going into ketosis too quickly. You may be impatient and want to jump into this plan with both feet, but I promise your odds of following through will greatly increase if you incorporate changes slowly. Many people are discouraged when they get the keto flu—your body's adverse reaction to low glucose levels and unbalanced electrolytes—and end up stopping the diet after only a few days. Begin slowly to allow a gentle introduction to ketosis.

One tool that is essential for monitoring your intake is a food tracker app (see the Resources on page 213 for suggestions). Start tracking your daily food and beverage intake from the beginning. I'd venture to say this will double your chances of success.

Step 1 (2 to 3 days): Stop eating all bread, sugar, desserts, sweets, and candy. Discontinue any regular sodas, juices, or beverages that have more than 1g of carbohydrate per serving.

Step 2 (2 to 3 days): Eliminate pasta, rice, and potatoes. At the same time, eat vegetables at each meal and increase your fat intake if this is particularly low. Don't be afraid of fat.

Step 3 (2 to 3 days): Discontinue all fruit with the exception of berries.

If you need a bit longer, please continue with this gentle carb elimination. If not, proceed to Week Two and let's get ketotic.

WEEKLY MIGRAINE DIARY

Fill out this worksheet at the end of Week One to check your overall progress and improve your ability to discover previously unknown triggers.

How many migraines did you suffer this week?

....

What time did the migraines start?

....

How long did the migraines last?

....

Did you do anything to treat them? Did it work?

....

What were you doing leading up to the attacks?

....

How was your overall sleep this week?

....

Did you notice any triggers or peaks after any meal this week?

....

Remember that for any of the meals this week, prepping ahead is a great idea. If you know you have a busy week, consider taking Sunday night to precook one or two meats for the week. Roast a pound of chicken breasts or thighs or pork chops and place them in the refrigerator to use for the next few days. Then all you have to do is add a vegetable and fat, and you're set. If you have a busy schedule, this will be essential to your success.

Remember to track your food intake online each day and shoot for a daily ketogenic ratio of between 1:1 and 2:1 and the macros mentioned in chapter 1.

Here are some other tips for the next three weeks:

Substitutions: It's always fine to trade olive oil for avocado or macadamia nut oils if you prefer a milder flavor.

Eat the fat: Make sure you eat *all* of the fat in these recipes—even the oil used in cooking.

Salad greens: These are very low in carbs. Up to 3 to 4 cups per day is not unreasonable. Please use greens as a way to get plenty of oil/fat into your diet by topping them with a tablespoon or two of low-carb dressing plus 1 to 2 tablespoons of olive oil or avocado oil.

Vegetables: When you see "+ vegetables" as part of a meal, feel free to choose any of the low-carb vegetables included in the ingredients lists of the recipes, or other vegetables with less than 5g total carbohydrates per cup. To keep the meal ketogenic, add 2 tablespoons of olive oil, avocado oil, butter, or a combination of these.

WEEK TWO SHOPPING LIST

For pantry items and dried herbs and spices, where I haven't specified a quantity, just buy a bottle, jar, bag, or pack. You'll be using them in the weeks and months ahead.

ANIMAL PROTEINS

- Beef chuck roast, 2 pounds
- Beef rib eye steaks, bone-in, 2 (¾-pound each)
- Pork belly, 1½ pounds, boneless
- Chicken breasts, 1 pound
- Roasting chicken, 1 (about 3 pounds)
- Turkey, ground, ¾ pound
- Eggs, large, 20

DAIRY

- Butter, 1 pound (sticks, grass-fed preferred)
- Cheddar cheese, full-fat, 8 ounces
- Cream cheese, full-fat, 12 ounces
- Goat cheese, full-fat, ½ cup
- Heavy (whipping) cream, 8 ounces
- Sour cream, 1 cup

PRODUCE

- Avocados, 2 (or more, always fine for a snack)
- Blueberries, 1 cup
- Boston lettuce, 1 head
- Cantaloupe, 1 small
- Cauliflower, 2 medium heads or 2 pounds cauliflower rice
- Celery, 1 bunch
- Cucumbers, 2
- Fennel, 1 small bulb
- Garlic, 2 heads (or a large jar of minced garlic)
- Jalapeño peppers, 3
- Kale, 1 small bunch
- Lemons, 2
- Limes, 2
- Mushrooms, 4 cups
- Onions, 3
- Raspberries, fresh or frozen, ½ cup
- Red bell peppers, 2
- Salad greens, 2 cups
- Scallions, 3
- Spinach, 5 cups
- Zucchini, 1

HERBS AND SPICES

- Basil, fresh, 1 bunch
- Black pepper
- Chipotle chili powder
- Cilantro, fresh, 1 bunch
- Cinnamon, ground
- Cumin, ground
- Nutmeg, ground
- Oregano, dried
- Parsley, fresh, 1 bunch
- Sea salt
- Thyme, fresh, 1 bunch

PANTRY ITEMS

- Almond butter, small jar
- Almond flour, 2-pound bag
- Almond meal, 1-pound bag
- Apple cider vinegar
- Avocado oil
- Beef stock, low-sodium, 6 cups
- Chia seeds, small bag
- Cocoa butter, large jar
- Coconut milk, canned, full-fat, 16 ounces
- Coconut oil, 16 ounces or more (great to use whenever fat is needed)
- Dijon mustard, small jar
- Macadamia nut oil (not required, but milder flavor and may be used in place of olive oil at any time)
- Macadamia nuts, 6 ounces (or lots more for the perfect snack)
- Mayonnaise, full-fat, 1 jar (or make your own Easy Mayonnaise, page 205)
- Olive oil (will use frequently; consider a light or mild flavored oil if you are not accustomed to the taste of olive oil)
- Pecans, ½ cup
- Protein powder, unsweetened vanilla, small can
- Salad dressing, full-fat Ranch or Italian (or make your own Green Goddess, page 201)
- Sliced almonds, ½ cup

- Soy sauce, small bottle (choose a brand with no MSG)
- Sriracha hot sauce, small jar
- Sweetener, erythritol-stevia blend such as Swerve, small bag (packets are fine)

- Tomato paste, no-salt-added, 6 ounces
- Tuna fish, water-packed, 1 can or pouch
- Unsweetened cocoa powder, small container
- Vanilla extract

OTHER
- Unsweetened shredded coconut, 1½ cups

WEEK TWO MEAL PLAN

	BREAKFAST	LUNCH	SNACK	DINNER
M	Creamy Kale Raspberry Smoothie (page 55)	Chicken Melon Salad (page 71)	1 to 2 ounces macadamia nuts	Roast Chicken with Cilantro Mayonnaise (page 163)
T	Almond Cream Cheese Pancakes with Blueberries (page 60)	Grilled chicken salad on "Quick and Dirty Meals" page 48, with Green Goddess Dressing (page 201)	Cinnamon Coconut Fat Bomb (page 95)	Turkey Pilaf (page 168)
W	Quick and Dirty Omelet (page 48)	Leftover Turkey Pilaf	Avocado Deviled Eggs (page 88)	Sriracha Pork Belly (page 174) + vegetable + 2 to 3 tablespoons fat
TH	Green Vanilla Smoothie (page 54)	Texas Style Beef Chili (page 119)	Cinnamon Coconut Fat Bomb	Spicy Pork Wraps (page 175)
F	Mushroom Cream Cheese Omelet (page 58)	Tuna wraps**	1 to 2 ounces macadamia nuts	Butter-Basted Rib Eye Steaks (page 179) + Simple Cauliflower Rice (page 96)
SAT	Leftover Mushroom Cream Cheese Omelet	Leftover Butter-Basted Rib Eye Steaks + Simple Cauliflower Rice	Cinnamon Coconut Fat Bomb	Chicken Cutlets with Garlic Cream Sauce (page 165) + vegetable + 2 to 3 tablespoons fat
SUN	Creamy Kale Raspberry Smoothie (page 55)	Leftover Chicken Cutlets with Garlic Cream Sauce	1 to 2 ounces macadamia nuts or Cinnamon Coconut Fat Bomb	Leftovers—finish anything left and start fresh tomorrow!

*Salad greens + 1 cup raw veggies + 2 to 3 ounces leftover chicken + 2 tablespoons avocado oil + 2 tablespoons Green Goddess Dressing

**1 can tuna, 2 to 3 tablespoons mayonnaise, chopped onions, and celery. Mix and use lettuce as the wrap.

WEEKLY MIGRAINE DIARY

Fill out this worksheet at the end of Week Two to check your overall progress and improve your ability to discover previously unknown triggers.

How many migraines did you suffer this week?

....

What time did the migraines start?

....

How long did the migraines last?

....

Did you do anything to treat them? Did it work?

....

What were you doing leading up to the attacks?

....

How was your overall sleep this week?

....

Did you notice any triggers or peaks after any meal this week?

....

SHOPPING TIPS

Here are some ideas for making grocery runs easier:

MAKE A LIST: Plan out your meals and snacks for four to seven days.

STICK TO THE LIST: Don't wind up with a cart full of items you don't need.

SHOP ONLINE: Imagine the time and energy you will save by just picking up your prepacked order or having it delivered.

WATCH NUTRITION LABELS: You are aiming for a 1:1 to 2:1 ketogenic ratio for each meal. Subtract the fiber from the total carbohydrates on a product to get the net carbs you will use to figure the ratio.

KEEP IN MIND TOTAL CARBOHYDRATES: A label that says "less than 1 gram of carbohydrate" could mean up to 0.99g of carbs. These seemingly insignificant carbs can add up and inhibit ketosis.

This week should be a little easier. You should be getting into the groove of cooking if this is new to you. Are you tracking your foods online yet? If not, I highly encourage you to start. This is an essential part of beginning to understand the carbohydrate, fat, and protein content of foods and getting your body into ketosis.

WEEK THREE SHOPPING LIST

This list assumes you already have the pantry items and dried spices from last week's list. They are appearing again on this week's menu.

ANIMAL PROTEINS

- Beef, ground, 1 pound
- Chicken breasts, 22 ounces
- Eggs, large, 12
- Lamb, ground, 1 pound
- Salmon fillets, 8 ounces
- Sausages, 2 (4 ounces each)
- Sea scallops, 12 ounces
- Shrimp, 8 ounces
- Tuna, raw, 4 ounces

DAIRY

- Butter, 1 stick
- Cheddar cheese, full-fat, ½ cup
- Cream cheese, full-fat, 30 ounces
- Goat cheese, full-fat, 8 ounces
- Gouda cheese, full-fat, 1 cup
- Heavy (whipping) cream, 2½ cups
- Jalapeño Cheddar cheese, full-fat, ¼ cup
- Mascarpone cheese, full-fat, ½ cup
- Parmesan cheese, ½ cup

PRODUCE

- Asparagus, 10 to 12 stalks
- Avocados, 2
- Bok choy, 3 baby heads
- Cabbage, 1 small head
- Cauliflower, 4 medium heads
- Celery, 1 head
- English cucumber, 1
- Fennel, 1 small bulb
- Garlic, 2 heads (or a large jar of minced garlic)
- Ginger, fresh, 2-inch piece
- Green bell pepper, 1
- Jalapeño pepper, 1
- Jicama, 1
- Kale, 2 large bunches
- Leeks, 3
- Lemons, 2
- Limes, 2
- Mixed greens, 6 cups
- Mushrooms, 3 cups
- Onions, 5
- Red onion, 1 small

- Red bell peppers, 4
- Scallions, 3
- Spaghetti squash, 1 small
- Spinach, 6 cups

- Strawberries, 1 cup
- Watercress, 1 small bunch
- Yellow bell pepper, 1

HERBS AND SPICES

- Basil, fresh, 1 bunch
- Basil, dried
- Cayenne pepper
- Chili powder
- Cilantro, fresh, 1 bunch
- Cloves, ground
- Coriander, ground
- Cumin, ground
- Fennel seeds

- Mint leaves, fresh, 1 bunch
- Oregano, fresh, 1 bunch
- Paprika, smoked
- Parsley, fresh, 1 bunch
- Red pepper flakes
- Southwest seasoning
- Thyme, fresh, 1 bunch
- Turmeric, ground

PANTRY ITEMS

- Cacao powder, small container
- Chicken stock, low-sodium, 10 cups
- Coconut milk, canned, full-fat, 7½ cups
- Hemp hearts, small package
- Liquid coffee extract, small bottle

- Mixed nuts, 1 ounce (great for snacking too)
- Nutritional yeast, small package
- Olive oil spray
- Thai red curry paste, small jar

OTHER

- Firm tofu, 6 ounces

WEEK THREE MEAL PLAN

	BREAKFAST	LUNCH	SNACK	DINNER
M	Simple Lamb Sausage (page 57) + 1 to 2 fried eggs (fry with lots of butter)	Chicken, Leek, and Cauliflower Soup (page 74) (make a day ahead)	Roasted Red Pepper Dip (page 84) with veggies	Roasted Spaghetti Squash Casserole (page 128)
T	Cabbage Sausage Hash Browns (page 59)	Leftover Chicken, Leek, and Cauliflower Soup	Creamy Tiramisu Fat Bomb (page 94)	Sea Scallops with Curry Sauce (page 154) + Simple Cauliflower Rice (page 96)
W	Leftover Cabbage Sausage Hash Browns	Leftover Sea Scallops with Curry Sauce + Simple Cauliflower Rice	Roasted Red Pepper Dip with veggies	White Chili (page 112)
TH	Strawberry Cheesecake Smoothie (page 56)	Leftover White Chili	Creamy Tiramisu Fat Bomb	Southwest Meatloaf with Lime Guacamole (page 176) + vegetables + 2 to 3 tablespoons fat
F	Mushroom Cream Cheese Omelet (page 58)	Tuna and Jicama Salad with Mint Cucumber Dressing (page 69)	Roasted Red Pepper Dip with veggies	Dark Leafy Green and Fresh Herb Soup (page 72) + Leftover Southwest Meatloaf with Lime Guacamole
SAT	Asparagus Gouda Frittata (page 61)	Leftover Dark Leafy Green and Fresh Herb Soup + 2 ounces mixed nuts	Triple Cheese Chips (page 86)	Seafood Coconut Stew (page 105)
SUN	Leftover Asparagus Gouda Frittata	Leftover Seafood Coconut Stew	Triple Cheese Chips	Leftover anything!

WEEKLY MIGRAINE DIARY

Fill out this worksheet at the end of Week Three to check your overall progress and improve your ability to discover previously unknown triggers.

How many migraines did you suffer this week?

....

What time did the migraines start?

....

How long did the migraines last?

....

Did you do anything to treat them? Did it work?

....

What were you doing leading up to the attacks?

....

How was your overall sleep this week?

....

Did you notice any triggers or peaks after any meal this week?

....

I hope by now you have more energy, think more clearly, are sleeping better and having fewer migraines!

You're going to love the meals this week—there are so many new recipes to try!

WEEK FOUR SHOPPING LIST

Once again, you already have many of the pantry items and dry spices for the week, as well as salad dressing and mayonnaise, so I have not added them to your shopping list. Make sure you haven't run out of olive oil, coconut oil, almond flour, and almond meal.

ANIMAL PROTEINS

- Beef chuck roast, 2 pounds
- Beef rib eye steak, boneless, 1 pound
- Beef, ground, ½ pound
- Eggs, large, 16
- Lamb, ground, 1 pound
- Pork rib chops, 4 (4 ounces each)
- Salmon, 12 ounces
- Sausages, 2 (4 ounces each)
- Turkey, ground, 1 pound

DAIRY

- Butter, 2 sticks
- Cheddar cheese, full-fat, 1¼ cups
- Cream cheese, full-fat, 8 ounces
- Hard cheese, full-fat, any variety, 2 ounces
- Heavy (whipping) cream, 2 cups
- Mascarpone cheese, full-fat, ½ cup
- Plain Greek yogurt, full-fat, 1 cup
- Sour cream, 2½ cups

PRODUCE

- Avocados, 6
- Blueberries, 1 cup
- Broccoli, 2 heads
- Brussels sprouts, 1 pound
- Cabbage, 1 small head
- Cantaloupe, 1 small
- Celery, 1 head
- Cucumber, 1
- English cucumbers, 2
- Garlic, 2 heads (or a large jar of minced garlic)
- Ginger, 1-inch piece
- Green bell pepper, 1
- Jalapeño peppers, 3
- Kale, 1 cup
- Lemons, 4
- Lettuce, 1 head
- Limes, 3

- Mushrooms, 4 cups
- Onions, 3
- Raspberries, ½ cup (fresh or frozen)
- Red bell peppers, 2
- Red onions, 2

- Scallions, 3
- Spinach, 2 cups
- Yellow zucchini, 2
- Zucchini, 2

HERBS AND SPICES

- Basil, fresh, 1 bunch
- Chipotle chili powder
- Cilantro, fresh, 1 bunch
- Garlic powder

- Oregano, fresh, 1 bunch
- Parsley, fresh, 1 bunch
- Thyme, fresh, 1 bunch

PANTRY ITEMS

- Beef stock, low-sodium, 6 cups
- Brazil nuts, ½ cup
- Chicken stock, low-sodium, 1 cup
- Cocoa butter, 2 tablespoons
- Coconut flour, 1-pound bag

- Coconut milk, canned, full-fat, 3 cups
- Macadamia nuts, 1 ounce (or more!)
- Pumpkin seeds, ½ cup
- Tomato paste, no-salt-added, 4 ounces

OTHER

- Black olives, 4 ounces
- Firm tofu, 6 ounces
- Unsweetened shredded coconut, ½ cup

WEEK FOUR MEAL PLAN

	BREAKFAST	LUNCH	SNACK	DINNER
M	Creamy Kale Raspberry Smoothie (page 55)	Shaved Brussels Sprouts Salad with Avocado Dressing (page 66)	Lime Almond Fat Bomb (page 91)	Texas Style Beef Chili (page 119)
T	Almond Cream Cheese Pancakes with Blueberries (page 60)	Leftover Texas Style Beef Chili + small salad	Taco Layer Dip (page 87)	Turkey Thyme Burgers (page 167) + Lemon Garlic Broccoli (page 97)
W	Leftover Almond Cream Cheese Pancakes with Blueberries + 1 egg scrambled with 1 tablespoon butter	Leftover Turkey Thyme Burgers + side salad with 2 tablespoons dressing + 1 tablespoon oil	Lime Almond Fat Bomb	"Fettuccini" with Avocado Alfredo (page 134)
TH	Green Vanilla Smoothie (page 54)	Leftover "Fettuccini" with Avocado Alfredo	Taco Layer Dip	Coconut Ginger Salmon Burgers (page 158) + Cold Cucumber and Avocado Soup (page 80)
F	Quick and Dirty Omelet (page 48)	Leftover Coconut Ginger Salmon Burgers + Cucumber Soup	Leftover Lime Almond Fat Bomb (page 91)	Pork Chops with Mushroom Sauce (page 172) + Grilled Cantaloupe (page 184)
SAT	Simple Lamb Sausage (page 57) + 1 egg scrambled with 1 tablespoon butter	Leftover Pork Chops with Mushroom Sauce + side salad	1 to 2 ounces macadamia nuts + 1 ounce hard cheese	Beef Fajitas (page 177) + Lime Guacamole (page 206)
SUN	Cabbage Sausage Hash Browns (page 59)	Leftover Beef Fajitas + Lime Guacamole	Lime Almond Fat Bomb	Leftover anything!

WEEKLY MIGRAINE DIARY

Fill out this worksheet at the end of Week Four to check your overall progress and improve your ability to discover previously unknown triggers.

How many migraines did you suffer this week?

....

What time did the migraines start?

....

How long did the migraines last?

....

Did you do anything to treat them? Did it work?

....

What were you doing leading up to the attacks?

....

How was your overall sleep this week?

....

Did you notice any triggers or peaks after any meal this week?

....

Adjust as Necessary

As you look through the recipes, you might see ingredients that could be a migraine trigger for you. Feel free to make reasonable adjustments as needed. Remember that the overall goal for every meal is to keep the ketogenic ratio intact. Fat: net carbs + protein.

Remember, to keep you in ketosis, I recommend an overall ratio of 1:1 to 2:1 for most adults, although some may need to push the fat a bit higher to achieve ketone levels high enough to affect some conditions. Also, remember to get enough salt in your new diet.

Keep this in mind as you make recipe substitutions. For instance, don't use whole milk instead of cream, because the milk's 12g of carbohydrates will drop you out of ketosis. You could use coconut cream instead. In general, be generous with fats and oils.

QUICK AND DIRTY MEALS

There are going to be days where you simply cannot use a formulated recipe—probably several times a week. Here's how to make a meal on those days.

PROTEIN + VEGETABLE + FAT

It's that simple:

- Choose a 2- to 4-ounce portion of protein.
- Add a low-carbohydrate vegetable (1 to 2 cups, or more for leafy greens)
- Add 2 to 3 tablespoons or more of oil, butter, mayonnaise, or heavy (whipping) cream

EXAMPLES

Grilled Chicken Salad: 2 to 3 cups green leaf lettuce, ½ cup raw vegetables, 3 ounces grilled chicken, 2 tablespoons ranch dressing, 2 tablespoons olive oil.

Bunless Burger: Combine a cooked 3-ounce hamburger patty (or a bratwurst), 3 tomato slices, lettuce, pickles, 1 slice onion, 2 tablespoons mayonnaise, 1 to 2 teaspoons mustard—and eat with a fork instead of a bun. To pair your burger with a drink, combine 2 tablespoons heavy (whipping) cream with unsweetened chocolate almond milk.

Quick and Dirty Omelet: Heat 2 tablespoons of butter in a skillet with ½ to 1 cup vegetables and sauté until done to your liking. Crack in 2 eggs, mix well to scramble, and cook until done. Top with 1 ounce of shredded Cheddar cheese.

Meat and Vegetables: Cook 3 ounces meat (any type) + 1 to 2 cups cauliflower rice (or other low-carb veggie) in 1 to 2 tablespoons olive oil + 1 to 2 tablespoons butter. Add garlic powder, onion powder, and salt, then 2 tablespoons heavy (whipping) cream.

Realistic Expectations

Chances are you have been fighting migraines for quite some time, enduring many ineffective treatments. Remember that every treatment—including this one—takes time. In general, when doctors prescribe a medication for a chronic condition, they'll tell you to come back in one, three, or six months. You have to go home, take your medicine, and wait. I wish I could tell you this was different, but it's not. You have to go home, cut the sugars, cut the carbs, increase the fat, get into ketosis . . . and wait.

How long? I've seen people improve in days, while for some it takes weeks. If you start and fail, start again. Most people are going to have some ups and downs. You might see some benefit and then fall off the wagon and have another migraine. Please don't lose heart.

I know one dietitian who tried a ketogenic diet for the migraines she had dealt with for 20 years. She had six to eight migraines per month, each lasting three to four days. After starting the diet, she went 14 weeks without a single migraine! She now has them only during weather changes. And here's a bonus: She no longer has acne, irritable bowel syndrome, joint pain, or thyroid issues. And, as an endurance runner, she is no longer experiencing "the wall."

Are these realistic expectations? Everyone will have a different story. What will yours be?

About the Recipes

I can't wait for you to try these recipes. There are many awesome, nutritious, flavor-filled dishes to make. Everyone will find something that appeals to their palate. If you love meat, we've got it: chicken cutlets, lamb chops, beef fajitas. Prefer seafood? No problem. Give the Sea Scallops with Curry Sauce (page 154) a try, or maybe the Salmon with Spinach Hemp Pesto (page 138).

Every aspect of your day is covered, from breakfast to dinner, soups to desserts. Not eating meat? Check out chapter 8, Meatless Mains. You'll find a lovely variety of main dishes featuring zucchini, cauliflower, spaghetti squash, and more.

Many of these recipes will take less than 30 minutes to prepare. If you're not accustomed to cooking that may seem like a long time, but in the big picture of what you're doing for your health, it's really not. Do I need to remind you how many hours you lose with each migraine?

Please enjoy the generous amounts of cream, butter, and oil included in these recipes. If your ketones aren't high enough, add a bit more fat to your meals.

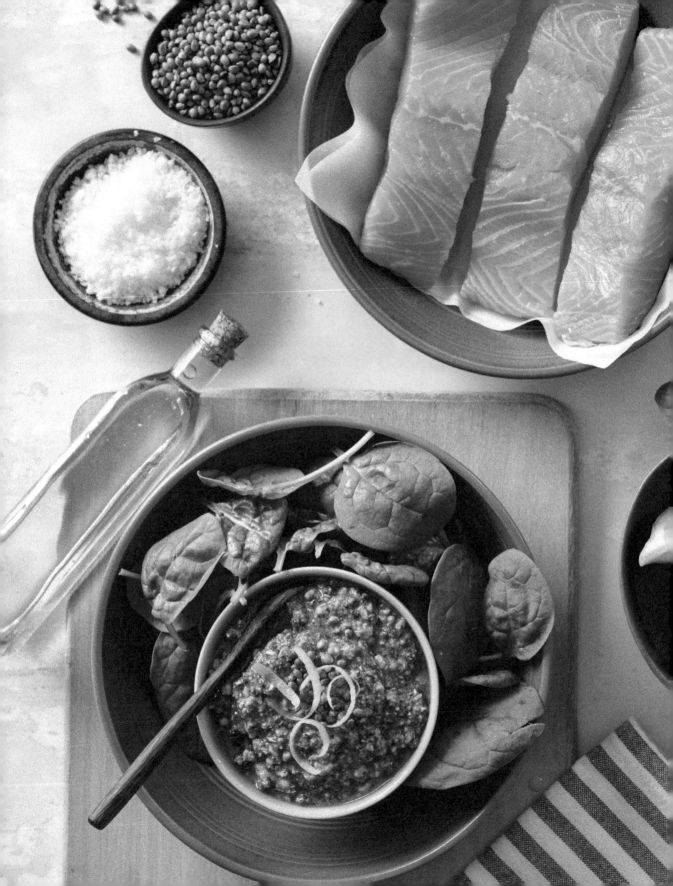

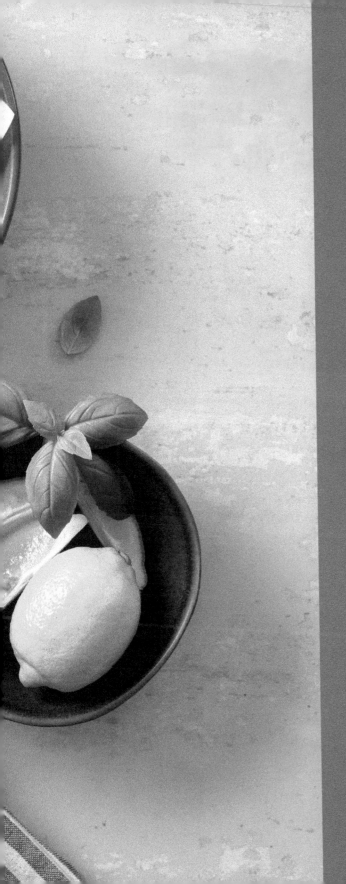

2

The
Recipes

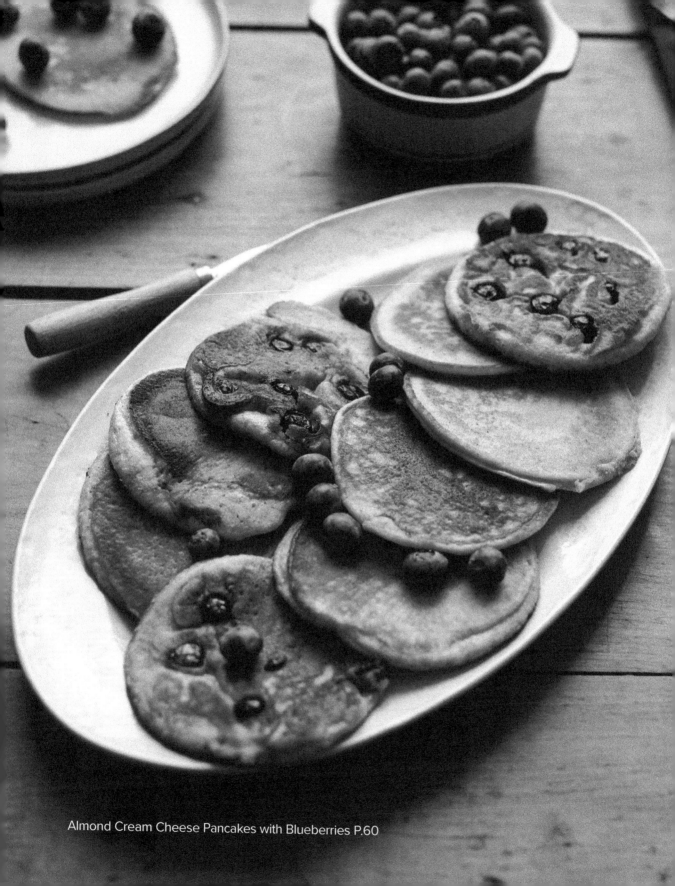

Almond Cream Cheese Pancakes with Blueberries P.60

CHAPTER 4

Breakfast

. . . .

Green Vanilla Smoothie

SERVES 2 / PREP TIME: 10 MINUTES

Smoothies can be the easiest, fastest choice to start your busy day
with lots of nutrients in one convenient glass. You can even take it
to go! Avocado, coconut milk, and chia seeds provide healthy fats
and omega fatty acids. *Chia* means "strength" in the ancient
Mayan language.

1 cup canned coconut milk
½ cucumber, cut into chunks
½ avocado
1 cup spinach
1 tablespoon chia seeds

1 scoop no-sugar-added vanilla
  protein powder
½ teaspoon ground cinnamon
½ teaspoon ground nutmeg
4 ice cubes

1. Put the coconut milk, cucumber, avocado, spinach, chia seeds, protein powder, cinnamon,
   and nutmeg in a blender.
2. Blend until the mixture is smooth and add the ice.
3. Blend until smooth and thick.
4. Pour the smoothie into 2 glasses and serve.

Make It Easy: A frozen diced avocado product works well in smoothies because you don't
have to worry about finding a ripe one in the produce section or storing the other half of the
unused fruit. If you use frozen, omit the ice cubes.

Per Serving
Macronutrients: Fat: 73 percent; Protein: 15 percent; Carbs: 12 percent
Ketogenic Ratio: 1.5:1
Calories: 382; Total Fat: 31g; Total Carbohydrates: 14g; Fiber: 7g;
Net Carbs: 7g; Protein: 14g; Sodium: 82mg; Sugar Alcohols: 0g

Creamy Kale Raspberry Smoothie

SERVES 2 / PREP TIME: 10 MINUTES

The heavy cream adds a luscious texture and makes the perfect base for sweet raspberries and leafy green kale. Kale is a wonderful choice for migraine sufferers because it is loaded with folate and magnesium. The kale provides almost 100mg of folate per smoothie portion.

1 cup kale

1 cup heavy (whipping) cream

½ cup frozen or fresh raspberries

½ teaspoon vanilla extract

¼ teaspoon ground cinnamon

2 ice cubes (4 if using fresh berries)

1. Place the kale, cream, raspberries, vanilla, and cinnamon in a blender.
2. Blend until thick and well mixed.
3. Add the ice cubes and blend until smooth.
4. Pour into 3 glasses and serve.

Substitution Tip: If you are lactose intolerant, swap out the heavy cream for canned coconut milk.

Per Serving
Macronutrients: Fat: 91 percent; Protein: 4 percent; Carbs: 5 percent
Ketogenic Ratio: 4.3:1
Calories: 425; Total Fat: 43g; Total Carbohydrates: 8g; Fiber: 2g;
Net Carbs: 6g; Protein: 4g Sugar Alcohols: 0g

Strawberry Cheesecake Smoothie

SERVES 4 / PREP TIME: 5 MINUTES

Fresh strawberries, tangy cream cheese, and coconut milk create a luscious dessert-like smoothie boosted with your favorite vanilla protein powder. Protein powder is a fabulous way to add this important nutrient to drinks and baked products, as long as you choose no-sugar-added powder to keep the carbs down.

1 cup halved strawberries

¼ cup chopped fennel

¾ cup cream cheese

1 cup canned coconut milk

1 scoop no-sugar-added vanilla protein powder

¼ teaspoon ground nutmeg

4 ice cubes

1. Put the strawberries, fennel, cream cheese, coconut milk, protein powder, and nutmeg in a blender.
2. Blend until the mixture is smooth.
3. Add the ice cubes and blend until thick and smooth.
4. Pour the mixture into 4 glasses and serve.

Substitution Tip: For extra berry flavor, try using a no-sugar-added strawberry protein powder instead of vanilla. If you're substituting the protein powder, add ½ teaspoon of vanilla extract to the smoothie mixture to enhance the taste.

Per Serving

Macronutrients: Fat: 79 percent; Protein: 12 percent; Carbs: 9 percent

Ketogenic Ratio: 1.7:1

Calories: 294; Total Fat: 26g; Total Carbohydrates: 7g; Fiber: 1g; Net Carbs: 6g; Protein: 9g; Sugar Alcohols: 0g

Simple Lamb Sausage

SERVES 4 / PREP TIME: 10 MINUTES / COOK TIME: 30 MINUTES

Hot, sizzling sausage served alongside a couple of sunny-side-up eggs is a hearty breakfast that can keep you full until lunch. The herb and spice combination in sausage is what makes each type taste special, from hot Italian to traditional bratwurst. Fennel seed is very common in Italian recipes, with its distinctive sweetish licorice-like taste.

1 pound ground lamb
½ onion, finely chopped
1 tablespoon chopped fresh parsley
2 teaspoons minced garlic
1 teaspoon dried basil
1 teaspoon paprika

¼ teaspoon sea salt
¼ teaspoon fennel seed
⅛ teaspoon freshly ground black pepper
Pinch ground cloves
2 tablespoons olive oil, divided

1. In a large bowl, stir together the lamb, onion, parsley, garlic, basil, paprika, salt, fennel seed, pepper, and cloves until very well mixed.
2. Divide the mixture into 8 equal portions and form them into ½-inch-thick patties.
3. Heat 1 tablespoon of olive oil in a large skillet over medium-high heat and panfry the patties 4 at a time, turning once, until cooked through and golden, about 15 minutes total.
4. Transfer the patties to a plate and repeat with the remaining patties and remaining olive oil.
5. Serve 2 patties per person.

Per Serving
Macronutrients: Fat: 78 percent; Protein: 20 percent; Carbs: 2 percent
Ketogenic Ratio: 1.7:1
Calories: 390; Total Fat: 34g; Total Carbohydrates: 2g; Fiber: 1g;
Net Carbs: 1g; Protein: 19g: Sugar Alcohols: 0g

Mushroom Cream Cheese Omelet

SERVES 2 / PREP TIME: 10 MINUTES / COOK TIME: 10 MINUTES

Shredded cheese is the usual filling for an omelet, but you may never go back to it after trying melted, rich chunks of cream cheese. Eggs are always a nutritious way to start your day because they contain protein, many vitamins, and essential fatty acids.

2 tablespoons butter, divided

2 cups sliced mushrooms

1 teaspoon minced garlic

4 eggs

⅛ teaspoon salt

Freshly ground black pepper

½ cup cream cheese, cubed

1 scallion, white and green parts, thinly sliced

1. Melt 1 tablespoon of butter in a large skillet over medium-high heat.
2. Sauté the mushrooms and garlic until lightly caramelized, about 5 minutes, and transfer to a plate.
3. Place the skillet back on the heat and melt the remaining butter.
4. In a medium bowl, whisk the eggs, salt, and pepper.
5. Pour the egg mixture into the skillet. As the eggs set, lift the edges of the omelet to allow the uncooked eggs to flow underneath. When the eggs are just set, with no liquid left on top, arrange the mushrooms on one side and top with chunks of cream cheese.
6. Fold the omelet in half and let stand for 1 minute to melt the cream cheese.
7. Cut in half and serve topped with scallion.

Substitution Tip: Try an assortment of wild mushrooms for an exotic taste. If using Portobello mushrooms, scoop out the black gills before sautéing or your eggs will turn gray.

Per Serving

Macronutrients: Fat: 79 percent; Protein: 16 percent; Carbs: 5 percent

Ketogenic Ratio: 1.7:1

Calories: 464; Total Fat: 41g; Total Carbohydrates: 6g; Fiber: 1g;

Net Carbs: 5g; Protein: 19g; Sugar Alcohols: 0g

Cabbage Sausage Hash Browns

SERVES 4 / PREP TIME: 10 MINUTES / COOK TIME: 10 MINUTES

Hash browns are usually made with potatoes or another starchy root vegetable fried to a golden brown, so cabbage might seem like an unusual choice. When you add sausage and egg to the cabbage, the mixture holds together well and this brassica vegetable crisps up nicely. Add a pinch red pepper flakes or chopped fresh oregano to boost the flavor and heat.

2 cups shredded cabbage
2 (4-ounce) cooked sausages or Simple Lamb Sausage (page 57) patties, chopped (8 ounces total)
2 eggs, beaten

½ onion, thinly sliced
1 teaspoon minced garlic
½ teaspoon chopped fresh thyme
2 tablespoons olive oil
Freshly ground black pepper

1. In a large bowl, stir together the cabbage, sausage, eggs, onion, garlic, and thyme and toss to combine.
2. Heat the olive oil in a large skillet over medium-high heat.
3. Divide the cabbage mixture into 4 equal patties and press them down with the flat of a spatula.
4. Cook until golden on the bottom, flip, and repeat with the other side, about 10 minutes total.
5. Season with pepper before serving.

Substitution Tip: Use Napa or green cabbage for the recipe instead of red cabbage. The recipe doesn't call for red cabbage.

Per Serving
Macronutrients: Fat: 75 percent; Protein: 19 percent; Carbs: 5 percent
Ketogenic Ratio: 1.5:1
Calories: 321; Total Fat: 27g; Total Carbohydrates: 4g; Fiber: 1g;
Net Carbs: 3g; Protein: 15g; Sugar Alcohols: 0g

Almond Cream Cheese Pancakes with Blueberries

SERVES 6 / PREP TIME: 10 MINUTES / COOK TIME: 12 MINUTES

Pancakes are like eating dessert for breakfast—a guilty pleasure
you usually have to abstain from when following a healthy diet.
But don't despair, these tender creations are nutritious, and
you would never guess the base is cheese.

1 cup almond flour

1 teaspoon Swerve

½ teaspoon ground cinnamon

¼ teaspoon ground nutmeg

1 cup cream cheese, at room temperature

5 eggs

½ teaspoon vanilla extract

3 tablespoons butter, divided

1 cup blueberries

1. In a large bowl, whisk together the almond flour, Swerve, cinnamon, and nutmeg.
2. In a medium bowl, whisk together the cream cheese, eggs, and vanilla.
3. Add the wet ingredients to the dry and whisk until smooth.
4. Melt 1 tablespoon of butter in a large skillet over medium heat.
5. Pour the batter into the skillet, about ¼ cup per pancake (about 4 per batch), and fry the pancakes until the bubbles on the top burst, about 2 minutes. Flip them over and fry until cooked through, about 4 minutes total.
6. Transfer to a plate and repeat in two more batches.
7. Serve 2 pancakes per person topped with blueberries.

Per Serving

Macronutrients: Fat: 81 percent; Protein: 13 percent; Carbs: 6 percent

Ketogenic Ratio: 1.7:1

Calories: 366; Total Fat: 33g; Total Carbohydrates: 10g; Fiber: 3g;
Net Carbs: 7g; Protein: 12g; Sugar Alcohols: <1g

Asparagus Gouda Frittata

SERVES 4 / PREP TIME: 10 MINUTES / COOK TIME: 12 MINUTES

Frittatas are crustless quiches, golden and bursting with vegetables, meats, and cheeses. This variation pairs buttery, mild Gouda with fresh asparagus and fragrant thyme for a spring-inspired meal. Gouda is rich in calcium, protein, vitamin B12, phosphorus, and zinc. There are 7 grams of protein per portion in this frittata from the cheese alone.

3 tablespoons butter, divided

½ onion, chopped

1 teaspoon minced garlic

2 cups asparagus, cut into 1-inch pieces

4 eggs

¼ teaspoon sea salt

⅛ teaspoon freshly ground black pepper

1 cup shredded mild Gouda cheese

2 tablespoons chopped fresh parsley

1. Preheat the oven to broil.
2. Melt half the butter in a medium ovenproof skillet over medium-high heat.
3. Sauté the onion and garlic until softened, about 3 minutes.
4. Stir in the asparagus and sauté until tender, about 4 minutes. Use a spoon to transfer the vegetables to a plate and take the skillet off the heat.
5. In a medium bowl, whisk together the eggs, salt, and pepper.
6. Return the skillet to the heat and melt the remaining butter.
7. Add the egg mixture to the skillet and cook until set, about 4 minutes, lifting the edges of cooked egg to allow the liquid to run underneath.

Continued on next page

8. When the eggs are just set, arrange the asparagus mixture evenly on top and top with cheese.
9. Transfer to the broiler and broil until the cheese is melted, about 1 minute.
10. Serve topped with parsley.

. . . .

Substitution Tip: If dairy is an issue, use coconut oil instead of butter and swap out the Gouda cheese for a vegan cheese of your choice. Using vegan cheese will drop the fat content slightly, so add an extra few teaspoons of oil to keep the ratio intact.

Per Serving

Macronutrients: Fat: 73 percent; Protein: 20 percent; Carbs: 7 percent

Ketogenic Ratio: 1.2:1

Calories: 271; Total Fat: 22g; Total Carbohydrates: 6g; Fiber: 2g;
Net Carbs: 4g; Protein: 15g; Sugar Alcohols: 0g

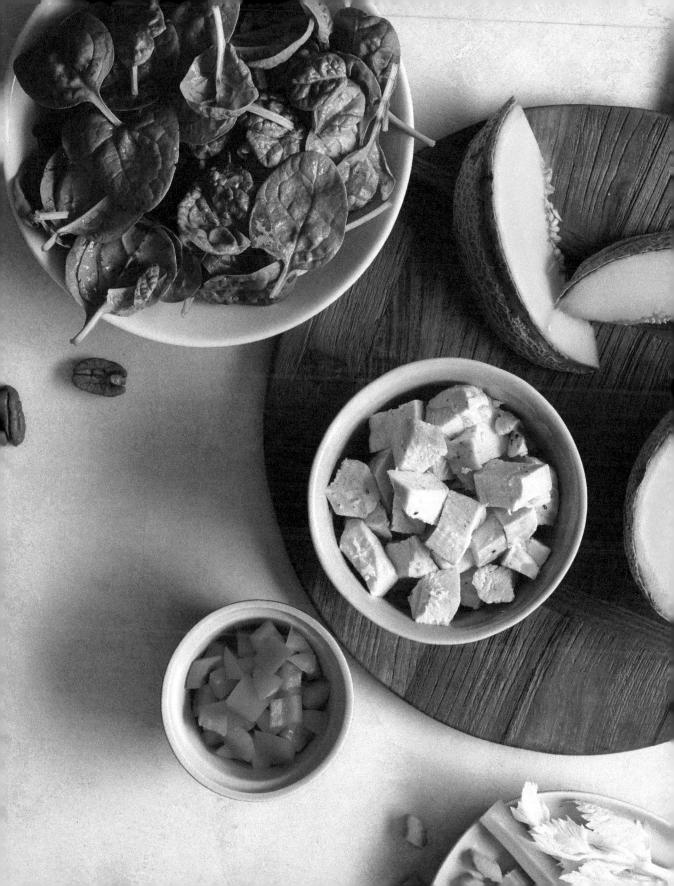

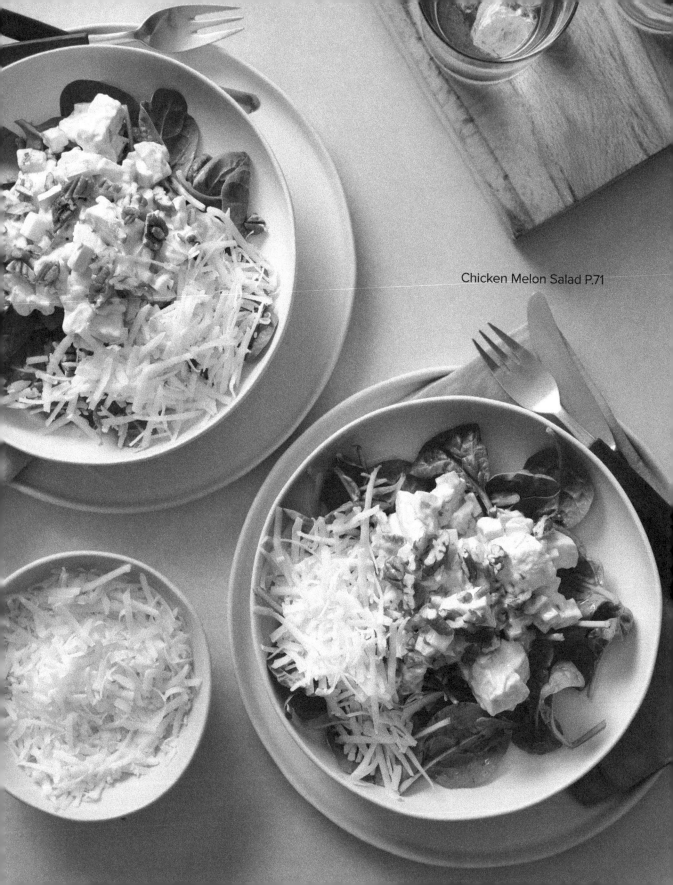

Chicken Melon Salad P.71

CHAPTER 5

Salads and Soups

. . . .

Shaved Brussels Sprouts Salad with Avocado Dressing

SERVES 4 / PREP TIME: 15 MINUTES

If you want a salad that's filling enough for a meal, look no further than this hearty recipe. Brussels sprouts are often overlooked brassica vegetables, taking a back seat to cauliflower, broccoli, and cabbage. But like their popular family members, Brussels sprouts are an incredible source of fiber.

FOR THE DRESSING

½ avocado

5 tablespoons olive oil

2 tablespoons chopped fresh cilantro

2 tablespoons freshly squeezed lemon juice

½ teaspoon minced garlic

Sea salt

Freshly ground black pepper

FOR THE SALAD

1 pound Brussels sprouts

4 hardboiled eggs, grated

¼ red onion, thinly sliced

¼ cup chopped fresh parsley

½ cup chopped Brazil nuts

TO MAKE THE DRESSING

1. Place the avocado, olive oil, cilantro, lemon juice, and garlic in a blender and pulse until smooth and thick.

2. Season with salt and pepper and set aside.

TO MAKE THE SALAD

1. Shave the Brussels sprouts into a large bowl using a mandoline or carrot peeler.
2. Add the eggs, red onion, and parsley and toss to combine.
3. Add the dressing and toss to coat.
4. Serve topped with Brazil nuts.

. . . .

Make It Easy: Wash the Brussels sprouts after you shave them because whole sprouts have a very tight cluster of leaves that can harbor dirt and grit.

Per Serving
Macronutrients: Fat: 79 percent; Protein: 15 percent; Carbs: 6 percent
Ketogenic Ratio: 1.8:1
Calories: 431; Total Fat: 38g; Total Carbohydrates: 15g; Fiber: 7g;
Net Carbs: 8g; Protein: 13g; Sugar Alcohols: 0g

Turkey and Kale Coleslaw

SERVES 4 / PREP TIME: 25 MINUTES

Coleslaw is a popular dish to serve at family events and potlucks because it's easy and inexpensive to make, and the crunchy vegetables bathed in tangy, sweet dressing are absolutely delicious. But coleslaw doesn't have to be just a side dish or topping. It can be a satisfying main meal when you add turkey and pumpkin seeds.

FOR THE DRESSING
1 cup heavy (whipping) cream
2 tablespoons apple cider vinegar
1 teaspoon freshly squeezed lemon juice
1 teaspoon Swerve
½ teaspoon ground cumin
¼ teaspoon sea salt

FOR THE SLAW
2 cups shredded Napa cabbage
1 cup shredded cooked turkey
1 cup shredded kale
1 cup shredded fennel
2 scallions, white and green parts, chopped
2 tablespoons chopped fresh parsley
½ cup toasted pumpkin seeds

TO MAKE THE DRESSING
1. In a small bowl, whisk together the cream, vinegar, lemon juice, Swerve, cumin, and salt.
2. Set aside.

TO MAKE THE SLAW
1. In a large bowl, toss together the cabbage, turkey, kale, fennel, scallions, and parsley.
2. Add the dressing and toss to coat.
3. Top with pumpkin seeds and serve.

Per Serving
Macronutrients: Fat: 70 percent; Protein: 19 percent; Carbs: 11 percent
Ketogenic Ratio: 1.1:1
Calories: 322; Total Fat: 25g; Total Carbohydrates: 11g; Fiber: 3g;
Net Carbs: 8g; Protein: 15g; Sugar Alcohols: 1g

Tuna and Jicama Salad with Mint Cucumber Dressing

SERVES 4 / PREP TIME: 20 MINUTES / COOK TIME: 10 MINUTES

Tuna salad usually conjures up mayonnaise-soaked fish pressed between two pieces of bread. But tuna can be elevated to become part of a pretty, nutritious salad that's perfect for a light dinner or lunch.

FOR THE DRESSING

1½ cups canned coconut milk

½ English cucumber, cut into chunks

¼ cup mint leaves

2 teaspoons freshly squeezed lemon juice

1 teaspoon Swerve

½ teaspoon ground coriander

FOR THE SALAD

2 tablespoons olive oil

¼ pound raw tuna fillet

4 cups mixed greens

1 jicama, peeled and shredded

3 baby bok choy, shredded

2 scallions, white and green parts, thinly sliced

½ cup crumbled goat cheese

TO MAKE THE DRESSING

1. Place the coconut milk, cucumber, mint, lemon juice, Swerve, and coriander in a blender and pulse until smooth.
2. Set aside.

TO MAKE THE SALAD

1. Heat the olive oil in a small skillet over medium-high heat.
2. Pan sear the tuna until it is just cooked through, turning once, about 10 minutes.
3. Chop the cooked tuna and set aside.
4. In a large bowl, toss together the mixed greens, jicama, and bok choy.

Continued on next page

5. Add three-quarters of the dressing to the salad and toss to coat.
6. Arrange the salad on four plates and top with the tuna, scallions, and goat cheese.
7. To serve, equally divide the remaining dressing between the plates, drizzling it over the top.

· ·

Nutrition Tip: Jicama is a juicy member of the bean family that's high in vitamins A, B, C, and K, as well as calcium, potassium, magnesium, and zinc.

Per Serving

Macronutrients: Fat: 65 percent; Protein: 17 percent; Carbs: 18 percent

Ketogenic Ratio: 1:1

Calories: 429; Total Fat: 31g; Total Carbohydrates: 21g; Fiber: 11g;
Net Carbs: 10g; Protein: 18g; Sugar Alcohols: 1g

Chicken Melon Salad

SERVES 3 / PREP TIME: 20 MINUTES

Simple is sometimes best, especially when you're tight on time and want a quick meal that still meets with your diet parameters. Sweet melon, crispy vegetables and greens, tasty chicken breast, and crunchy pecans create a sublime nutrient-packed meal. The vibrant chicken salad topping can also be spooned into lettuce leaves for a grab-and-go wrap.

4 ounces cooked boneless, skinless chicken breast, chopped
2 celery stalks, chopped
½ cup diced cantaloupe
½ red bell pepper, chopped
½ cup mayonnaise

1 tablespoon chopped basil
Sea salt
Freshly ground black pepper
4 cups baby spinach
1 cup shredded Cheddar cheese
½ cup chopped pecans

1. In a medium bowl, mix together the chicken, celery, cantaloupe, bell pepper, mayonnaise, and basil. Season the chicken salad with salt and pepper.
2. Arrange the baby spinach on three plates and top each with a generous scoop of chicken salad.
3. Top with cheese and pecans and serve.

Nutrition Tip: Spinach is exceptionally high in vitamins A and K, as well as manganese and folate.

Per Serving
Macronutrients: Fat: 81 percent; Protein: 14 percent; Carbs: 5 percent
Ketogenic Ratio: 1.9:1
Calories: 621; Total Fat: 56g; Total Carbohydrates: 12g; Fiber: 5g;
Net Carbs: 7g; Protein: 22g; Sugar Alcohols: 0g

Dark Leafy Green and Fresh Herb Soup

SERVES 4 / PREP TIME: 15 MINUTES / COOK TIME: 20 MINUTES

Dark leafy greens aren't just for salads—they are the perfect assertively flavored base for this creamy, herb-packed soup. The tofu and heavy cream create a thick, velvety texture and add healthy fats and protein to the meal. Tofu is packed with iron, calcium, and protein and can help reduce the risk of cardiovascular disease, type 2 diabetes, and cancer.

3 tablespoons avocado oil

1 onion, chopped

2 teaspoons minced garlic

4½ cups chopped spinach

4½ cups chopped kale

1¾ cups watercress

4 cups low-sodium chicken stock or Chicken Bone Broth (page 207)

6 ounces firm tofu, cut into cubes

2 tablespoons chopped fresh basil

1 tablespoon chopped fresh oregano

2 teaspoons chopped fresh thyme

1 cup heavy (whipping) cream

Sea salt

Freshly ground black pepper

1. Heat the oil in a large stockpot over medium-high heat.
2. Sauté the onion and garlic until tender, about 3 minutes.
3. Add the spinach, kale, watercress, and chicken stock and bring to a boil.

4. Reduce the heat to low and simmer the soup until the greens are tender, about 10 minutes.
5. Stir in the tofu, basil, oregano, and thyme, and simmer 5 minutes.
6. Transfer the soup to a food processor or use an immersion blender to purée the soup until it is very smooth.
7. Return the soup to the stockpot.
8. Whisk in the cream and season with salt and pepper. Serve immediately.

- -

Nutrition Tip: There is a very generous quantity of herbs in this delicious soup, so it is essential to use excellent-quality plants. Try to find organic herbs or use some from your own garden.

Per Serving
Macronutrients: Fat: 78 percent; Protein: 11 percent; Carbs: 11 percent
Ketogenic Ratio: 1.6:1
Calories: 406; Total Fat: 35g; Total Carbohydrates: 16g; Fiber: 5g;
Net Carbs: 11g; Protein: 11g; Sugar Alcohols: 0g

Chicken, Leek, and Cauliflower Soup

SERVES 4 / PREP TIME: 20 MINUTES / COOK TIME: 35 MINUTES

Hearty soups are fun to prepare and a fabulous way to fill up on a plethora of healthy, nutrient-rich ingredients all in one bowl. Don't let the simple title fool you—this is an elegant, complex soup consisting of a smooth, creamy cauliflower base studded with chunks of juicy chicken and topped with luscious goat cheese and fresh parsley. This recipe is great for using up leftover roast chicken or turkey.

3 tablespoons olive oil, divided

6 ounces boneless, skinless chicken breast, cut into ½-inch chunks

3 leeks, light green and white parts, chopped and washed

2 teaspoons minced garlic

1 medium head cauliflower, coarsely chopped

4 cups low-sodium chicken stock or Chicken Bone Broth (page 207)

1 cup heavy (whipping) cream

½ teaspoon ground nutmeg

Sea salt

Freshly ground black pepper

½ cup crumbled soft goat cheese

1 tablespoon chopped fresh parsley

1. Heat 2 tablespoons of olive oil in a large stockpot over medium-high heat.
2. Add the chicken and sauté until cooked through, about 10 minutes. With a slotted spoon, transfer the chicken to a plate.
3. Add the remaining olive oil to the stockpot.

4. Sauté the leeks and garlic until tender, about 5 minutes.
5. Add the cauliflower and chicken stock and bring the soup to a boil.
6. Reduce the heat to low and simmer until the vegetables are tender, about 20 minutes.
7. Transfer the soup to a food processor, or use an immersion blender, and purée the soup until very smooth.
8. Return the soup to the pot and whisk in the reserved chicken, cream, and nutmeg.
9. Season with salt and pepper.
10. Serve topped with goat cheese and parsley.

. . . .

Nutrition Tip: Heavy cream adds crucial fat to this soup as well as providing vitamins A, D, and B2 and phosphorus.

Per Serving
Macronutrients: Fat: 70 percent; Protein: 17 percent; Carbs: 13 percent
Ketogenic Ratio: 1:1
Calories: 477; Total Fat: 37g; Total Carbohydrates: 21g; Fiber: 5g;
Net Carbs: 16g; Protein: 20g; Sugar Alcohols: 0g

Hearty Lamb Cabbage Soup

SERVES 6 / PREP TIME: 15 MINUTES / COOK TIME: 35 MINUTES

If you have a little extra prep time, instead of sautéing the lamb at the beginning, roll the ground meat into 1-inch balls and throw them in at step 5 when the soup is simmering. Meatballs are fun to eat, and the lamb flavor will still infuse the broth. Don't leave out the bay leaves because they add an almost minty, slightly bitter flavor that can make the strong lamb taste less heavy.

3 tablespoons olive oil, divided

1 pound ground lamb

1 onion, chopped

2 celery stalks, chopped

2 teaspoons minced garlic

2 cups shredded green cabbage

6 cups low-sodium chicken stock or Chicken Bone Broth (page 207)

2 bay leaves

2 teaspoons chopped fresh thyme

Sea salt

Freshly ground black pepper

1. Heat 1 tablespoon of olive oil in a large saucepan over medium-high heat.
2. Sauté the lamb until cooked through, about 10 minutes, and transfer to a plate using a slotted spoon.
3. Add the remaining olive oil and sauté the onion, celery, and garlic until the vegetables are tender, about 3 minutes.
4. Add the cabbage, chicken stock, and bay leaves and bring the soup to a boil.
5. Reduce the heat to low and simmer until the cabbage is tender, about 15 minutes.
6. Add the cooked lamb and thyme and simmer until the lamb is heated through, about 5 minutes.
7. Remove the bay leaves and season the soup with salt and pepper to serve.

Per Serving

Macronutrients: Fat: 75 percent; Protein: 20 percent; Carbs: 5 percent

Ketogenic Ratio: 1.4:1

Calories: 300; Total Fat: 25g; Total Carbohydrates: 4g; Fiber: 1g; Net Carbs: 3g; Protein: 15g; Sugar Alcohols: 0g

Creamy Broccoli, Bacon, and Cheese Soup

SERVES 6 / PREP TIME: 15 MINUTES / COOK TIME: 30 MINUTES

This is not a delicate soup; it's creamy, cheesy, studded with bacon, and absolutely delicious. This soup is made in two stages, with a puréed broccoli base and tender florets added after blanching them separately. You can skip this step and purée everything together, but the florets add a lovely texture and visual impact to the soup. Look for nitrate-free uncured bacon at your meat counter in the local grocery store to avoid this common migraine trigger.

2 heads broccoli
2 tablespoons olive oil
1 onion, chopped
2 teaspoons minced garlic
4 cups low-sodium vegetable stock
½ teaspoon ground nutmeg

1 cup heavy (whipping) cream
Sea salt
Freshly ground black pepper
1 cup shredded Cheddar cheese
4 slices uncured bacon, cooked
  and chopped

1. Chop one head of broccoli, including the stem, and cut the remaining head into small florets and chop the stem. Set the florets aside.
2. Heat the olive oil in a large saucepan over medium-high heat.
3. Sauté the onion and garlic until tender, about 3 minutes.
4. Add the chopped broccoli, stock, and nutmeg.
5. Bring the soup to a boil, then reduce the heat to low and simmer until the vegetables are tender, about 25 minutes.
6. While the soup is simmering, place a medium pot of water over high heat and bring to a boil. Blanch the florets until tender-crisp, about 3 minutes, and drain.

Continued on next page

7. Transfer the soup to a food processor or use an immersion blender and blend until smooth, then transfer back to the saucepan.
8. Whisk in the cream and blanched florets.
9. Season with salt and pepper. Serve topped with cheese and bacon.

. . . .

Nutrition Tip: Onion adds more than flavor to this tempting soup. This allium provides prebiotic fiber which serves as food for probiotics in the gut.

Per Serving

Macronutrients: Fat: 82 percent; Protein: 13 percent; Carbs: 5 percent
Ketogenic Ratio: 2:1
Calories: 320; Total Fat: 29g; Total Carbohydrates: 7g; Fiber: 2g;
Net Carbs: 5g; Protein: 10g; Sugar Alcohols: 0g

Cream of Mushroom Soup

SERVES 4 / PREP TIME: 10 MINUTES / COOK TIME: 27 MINUTES

The richness and intense mushroom flavor of this dish might surprise you if canned soup is your go-to choice. Thyme and whipping cream create an elegant, sophisticated preparation, as well.

⅓ cup butter

8 ounces wild mushrooms

1 onion, chopped

2 teaspoons minced garlic

3 tablespoons almond flour

4 cups low-sodium chicken stock or Chicken Bone Broth (page 207)

1 cup heavy (whipping) cream

2 teaspoons chopped fresh thyme

Sea salt

Freshly ground black pepper

1. Melt the butter in a large saucepan over medium-high heat.
2. Sauté the mushrooms, onion, and garlic in the butter until lightly caramelized, stirring frequently, about 12 minutes.
3. Stir in the almond flour and then whisk in the chicken stock.
4. Heat the soup until it is thickened and hot but not boiling, about 15 minutes.
5. Whisk in the cream and thyme.
6. Transfer half the soup to a blender or food processor and purée. Then stir it back into the remaining soup.
7. Season with salt and pepper and serve.

Nutrition Tip: Thyme is very high in flavonoids and healthy volatile oils, as well as vitamins A, B6, C, and K.

Per Serving

Macronutrients: Fat: 88 percent; Protein: 6 percent; Carbs: 6 percent

Ketogenic Ratio: 3:1

Calories: 411; Total Fat: 40g; Total Carbohydrates: 9g; Fiber: 2g;

Net Carbs: 7g; Protein: 6g; Sugar Alcohols: 0g

Cold Cucumber and Avocado Soup

SERVES 4 / PREP TIME: 15 MINUTES

Cold soups might not be in your culinary repertoire yet, but they'll likely find a place after you dip your spoon into this pastel green soup. Fresh and creamy, with a hint of heat and tartness—it's completely addictive! Cucumber is a bright-tasting water-packed vegetable (about 96 percent water), so it can hydrate the body while pleasing the palate. Dehydration is one of the most common causes of headaches.

2 English cucumbers, cut into chunks

2 avocados, cubed

1 cup plain Greek yogurt

6 ounces firm tofu, diced

1 scallion, white and green parts, cut into chunks

Juice of 1 lemon

¼ jalapeño pepper

1 cup low-sodium chicken stock or Chicken Bone Broth (page 207)

2 tablespoons Spinach Hemp Pesto (page 204)

Sea salt

Freshly ground black pepper

½ cup mascarpone cheese

1. In a blender, purée the cucumber, avocados, yogurt, tofu, scallion, lemon juice, and jalapeño until very smooth.
2. Add the chicken stock and pesto and blend until you have the desired texture and thickness.
3. Season with salt and pepper and serve topped with mascarpone cheese.

Make It Easy: Make this soup the day before so that the flavors have time to mature and mellow. The lemon juice will keep the color from oxidizing and brighten the flavor.

Per Serving

Macronutrients: Fat: 75 percent; Protein: 10 percent; Carbs: 15 percent

Ketogenic Ratio: 1.6:1

Calories: 398; Total Fat: 33g; Total Carbohydrates: 18g; Fiber: 7g; Net Carbs: 11g; Protein: 10g; Sugar Alcohols: 0g

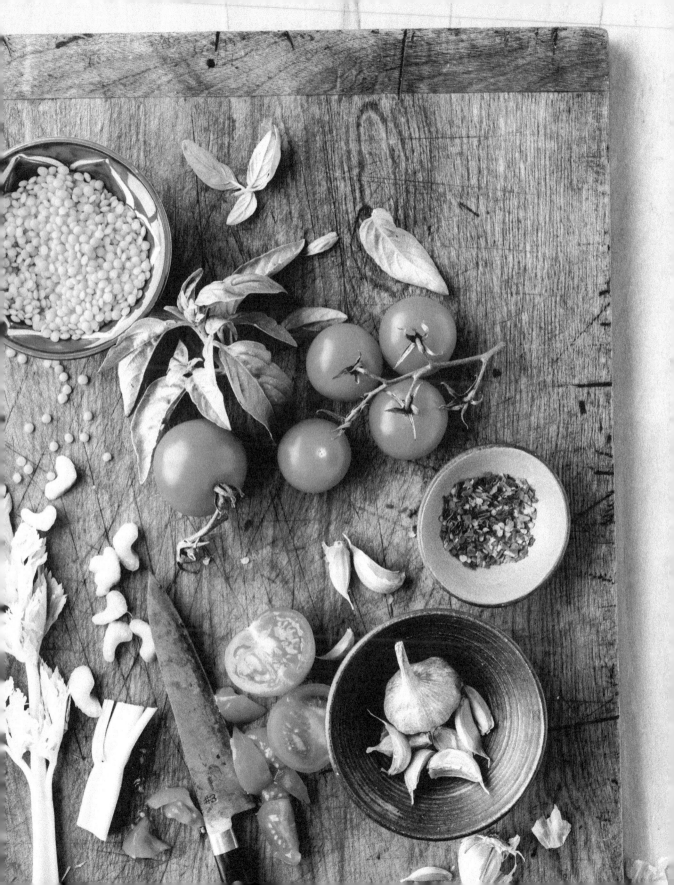

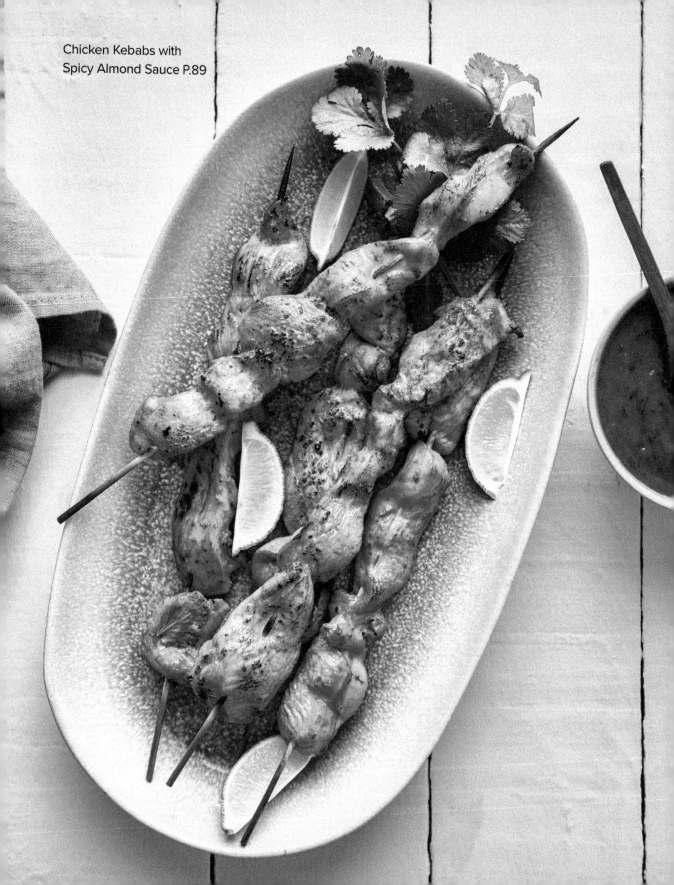

Chicken Kebabs with
Spicy Almond Sauce P.89

Snacks and Sides

Roasted Red Pepper Dip

SERVES 6 / PREP TIME: 20 MINUTES / COOK TIME: 6 MINUTES

Roasting red bell peppers creates a rich, smoky, fragrant flavor perfect for dips and other recipes, elevating an already delicious ingredient to new culinary heights. Double up this recipe and try tossing the dip with spiralized zucchini for a tasty "pasta" main course.

3 red bell peppers, halved
2 tablespoons melted coconut oil
1 cup cream cheese
2 tablespoons hemp hearts
2 tablespoons chopped fresh parsley

2 tablespoons chopped fresh basil
2 tablespoons freshly squeezed lemon juice
Pinch red pepper flakes
Sea salt
Freshly ground black pepper

1. Preheat the oven to broil.
2. Place the bell peppers on a baking tray and massage to coat with the coconut oil.
3. Broil them skin-side up until the peppers are tender and the skin is charred, about 6 minutes.
4. Let the peppers cool for 10 minutes and scrape off the skin.
5. Place the peppers, cream cheese, hemp hearts, parsley, basil, lemon juice, and red pepper flakes in a food processor or blender and pulse until smooth and creamy.
6. Season with salt and pepper.
7. Store the dip for up to 1 week in a sealed container in the refrigerator.

Make It Easy: Since it freezes well for up to 3 months in a sealed container, double the recipe. Thaw in the refrigerator overnight and stir before serving.

Per Serving
Macronutrients: Fat: 87 percent; Protein: 10 percent; Carbs: 3 percent
Ketogenic Ratio: 2.2:1
Calories: 208; Total Fat: 20g; Total Carbohydrates: 6g; Fiber: 2g;
Net Carbs: 4g; Protein: 5g; Sugar Alcohols: 0g

Sesame Meatballs

SERVES 8 / PREP TIME: 20 MINUTES / COOK TIME: 12 MINUTES

Sesame seeds and a splash of soy sauce create an exotic, juicy
meatball that's perfect as a main course or as a tempting appetizer.
You can even add a delicious dipping sauce, such as the one in the
Chicken Kebabs with Spicy Almond Sauce recipe (page 89).

1 pound ground beef
¼ cup almond flour
¼ cup sesame seeds
1 egg, beaten

1 scallion, white and green parts, chopped
1 tablespoon soy sauce
2 tablespoons olive oil

1. In a large bowl, combine the ground beef, almond flour, sesame seeds, egg, scallion, and
   soy sauce until well mixed.
2. Roll the beef mixture into 1-inch meatballs.
3. Heat the olive oil over medium heat in a large skillet.
4. Cook the meatballs until golden and cooked through, turning to brown all sides,
   10 to 12 minutes total.
5. Serve.

Nutrition Tip: Sesame seeds are very rich in vitamin E and add a lovely crunch to these
Asian-inspired meatballs.

Per Serving
Macronutrients: Fat: 77 percent; Protein: 23 percent; Carbs: 1 percent
Ketogenic Ratio: 1.4:1
Calories: 221; Total Fat: 19g; Total Carbohydrates: 2g; Fiber: 1g;
Net Carbs: 1g; Protein: 13g; Sugar Alcohols: 0g

Triple Cheese Chips

SERVES 4 / PREP TIME: 10 MINUTES / COOK TIME: 7 MINUTES

There's something almost magical about how heaps of shredded cheese turn into golden, crispy treats that are perfect as a snack or a salad topper for a special occasion. Look for fresh Parmesan cheese rather than aged, so you avoid migraine-causing tyramine. You can eliminate the Parmesan altogether and just use the Cheddars if you are particularly sensitive.

Olive oil spray
½ cup finely shredded Parmesan cheese
½ cup finely shredded Cheddar cheese

¼ cup finely shredded jalapeño Cheddar cheese
Pinch cayenne pepper

1. Preheat the oven to 425°F.
2. Lightly spray a baking sheet with oil and line with parchment paper.
3. In a medium bowl, toss together the Parmesan, Cheddars, and cayenne pepper until well mixed.
4. Drop the cheese mixture onto the baking sheet, about 1½ tablespoons per chip. Spread out the cheese with the back of a spoon, leaving a minimum of 1 inch between the edges.
5. Bake until melted and bubbly, but do not brown, 5 to 7 minutes.
6. Remove the chips from the baking sheet and cool on a baking rack.
7. Store in a sealed container at room temperature for up to 3 days.

Make It Easy: You can use a packaged shredded cheese product instead of grating everything yourself. There are many different blends in the grocery store.

Per Serving
Macronutrients: Fat: 72 percent; Protein: 29 percent; Carbs: 1 percent
Ketogenic Ratio: 1:1
Calories: 138; Total Fat: 11g; Total Carbohydrates: 1g; Fiber: 0g;
Net Carbs: 1g; Protein: 10g; Sugar Alcohols: 0g

Taco Layer Dip

SERVES 6 / PREP TIME: 20 MINUTES / COOK TIME: 20 MINUTES

Yes, you can make a traditional seven-layer dip without the legumes or tortilla chips. This creation is still seven layers if you count the fresh cilantro topping. Serve this dip with raw vegetables.

1 tablespoon olive oil
½ pound ground beef
1 tablespoon chili powder
2 teaspoons ground cumin
1 teaspoon paprika
½ teaspoon garlic powder

1 red bell pepper, chopped
½ red onion, chopped
½ cup chopped black olives
1 cup shredded Cheddar cheese
1 cup sour cream
1 tablespoon chopped fresh cilantro

1. Preheat the oven to 400°F.
2. Heat the olive oil in a large skillet and brown the ground beef until cooked through, about 10 minutes.
3. Stir in the chili powder, cumin, paprika, and garlic powder.
4. Spread the ground beef in a 9-by-13-inch casserole dish and top with bell pepper, red onion, black olives, and Cheddar cheese.
5. Bake in the oven until the cheese is bubbly and melted, about 10 minutes.
6. Top with sour cream and cilantro and serve.

Substitution Tip: If nightshades are a concern because of a FODMAPs sensitivity or autoimmune condition, omit the red bell pepper and the paprika from this dip. Try finely chopped cauliflower instead.

Per Serving
Macronutrients: Fat: 73 percent; Protein: 16 percent; Carbs: 11 percent
Ketogenic Ratio: 1.3:1
Calories: 319; Total Fat: 26g; Total Carbohydrates: 8g; Fiber: 1g;
Net Carbs: 7g; Protein: 13g; Sugar Alcohols: 0g

Avocado Deviled Eggs

SERVES 4 / PREP TIME: 20 MINUTES

Deviled eggs are still trendy cocktail party fare, but the roots of this stuffed egg stretch back to ancient Rome, where seasoned sauce-stuffed eggs were the main course. This version has a Southwest flair with avocado, jalapeño pepper, lime, and cilantro. The combination with the yolks creates a pastel green filling flecked with darker green. If you like different flavor combinations, try curry, sundried tomato, pesto, and traditional mayonnaise fillings.

6 hardboiled eggs
½ ripe avocado
1 tablespoon freshly squeezed lime juice

1 teaspoon minced fresh cilantro
1 teaspoon minced jalapeño pepper
Sea salt

1. Peel the hardboiled eggs and carefully cut them in half lengthwise.
2. Remove the yolks and set them aside in a small bowl.
3. Mash the egg yolks, avocado, lime juice, cilantro, and jalapeño until well combined and creamy.
4. Season with salt.
5. Spoon the yolk mixture into the center of the egg whites, distributing evenly, and serve.

Make It Easy: Do not hard-boil extremely fresh eggs or you will have a hard time removing the shell. Older eggs are best. Also, shock your newly boiled eggs in very cold water to stop the cooking process, so you do not get unsightly dark rings around the yolks.

Per Serving
Macronutrients: Fat: 64 percent; Protein: 26 percent; Carbs: 10 percent
Ketogenic Ratio: 1:1
Calories: 155; Total Fat: 11g; Total Carbohydrates: 3g; Fiber: 2g;
Net Carbs: 1g; Protein: 10g; Sugar Alcohols: 0g

Chicken Kebabs with Spicy Almond Sauce

SERVES 4 / PREP TIME: 15 MINUTES, PLUS TIME TO MARINATE / COOK TIME: 12 MINUTES

Kebabs are simply marinated or seasoned meat skewered on sticks and broiled or grilled. A spicy or savory sauce usually accompanies these juicy kebabs. Chicken is used in this recipe, but you can also try beef, pork, sea scallops, lamb, or traditional ox tongue. The almond butter sauce will work with all these variations.

FOR THE ALMOND BUTTER SAUCE

½ cup almond butter

1 tablespoon soy sauce

1 tablespoon finely chopped fresh cilantro

1 teaspoon Swerve

1 teaspoon minced garlic

Juice of 1 lime

Pinch red pepper flakes

FOR THE KEBABS

Juice of 1 lime

¼ cup olive oil

2 tablespoons soy sauce

1 tablespoon minced garlic

¾ pound boneless, skinless chicken breast cut into strips

TO MAKE THE ALMOND BUTTER SAUCE

1. Whisk together the almond butter, soy sauce, cilantro, Swerve, garlic, lime juice, and red pepper flakes in a small bowl until well combined.
2. Set aside, covered, in the refrigerator.

TO MAKE THE KEBABS

1. In a medium bowl, stir together the lime juice, olive oil, soy sauce, garlic, and chicken until well mixed.
2. Marinate at least 1 hour and up to 24 hours, covered, in the refrigerator.
3. Preheat the oven to broil.
4. Remove the chicken strips from the marinade and thread them onto wooden skewers that have been soaked in water.

Continued on next page

5. Arrange the kebabs on a baking sheet and broil, turning once, until the meat is cooked through but still juicy, 10 to 12 minutes total.
6. Serve with almond butter sauce.

- -

Substitution Tip: Use peanut butter or other nut butters to make this very rich sauce if allergies are not a concern. Use the other nut butters in the same amount as the almond butter.

Per Serving
Macronutrients: Fat: 73 percent; Protein: 22 percent; Carbs: 5 percent
Ketogenic Ratio: 1.1:1
Calories: 409; Total Fat: 33g; Total Carbohydrates: 9g; Fiber: 3g;
Net Carbs: 6g; Protein: 23g; Sugar Alcohols: 1g

Lime Almond Fat Bomb

MAKES 16 / PREP TIME: 20 MINUTES, PLUS TIME TO CHILL / COOK TIME: 2 MINUTES

These tasty treats contain a double serving of almonds, in the bomb itself and as a coating. Lime zest and juice add a delightful tartness that's offset by a little sweetener. Almonds are very high in magnesium, which can be important because migraine sufferers often have low levels of this mineral. One ounce of almonds has about 80mg of magnesium, so try to include them regularly in your diet if nuts are not an issue.

½ cup coconut oil
2 tablespoons cocoa butter
Juice and zest of 1 lime
½ teaspoon vanilla extract

½ cup coconut flour
½ cup almond flour
1 teaspoon Swerve
½ cup almond meal

1. In a small saucepan over medium heat, stir together the coconut oil, cocoa butter, lime juice, lime zest, and vanilla until the mixture is smooth and melted, about 2 minutes.
2. Remove from the heat and set aside.
3. In a medium bowl, stir together the coconut flour, almond flour, and Swerve until well combined.
4. Add in the coconut oil mixture and stir until well blended.
5. Place the bowl in the refrigerator until firm enough to form into balls, about 1 hour.

Continued on next page

6. Roll the fat bombs into balls and roll them in the almond meal to coat.
7. Place the balls in the freezer in a sealed container until very firm, about 3 hours.
8. Serve frozen. Store in the freezer for up to 1 month in a sealed container.

. . . .

Substitution Tip: Almond meal and almond flour might seem the same, but there is a distinct texture difference. Flour is finer and is used as a great baking substitute for wheat flour. Meal is coarser, sometimes with small bits of almonds, and has more texture.

Per Serving

Macronutrients: Fat: 83 percent; Protein: 6 percent; Carbs: 11 percent
Ketogenic Ratio: 3:1
Calories: 130; Total Fat: 12g; Total Carbohydrates: 4g; Fiber: 2g;
Net Carbs: 2g; Protein: 2g; Sugar Alcohols: 1g

Avocado Chili Fat Bomb

MAKES 10 / PREP TIME: 25 MINUTES, PLUS TIME TO CHILL

Many fat bomb recipes are quite sweet, as they're often packed with coconut and nut butter, so it's nice to have another option in the freezer for those moments when a savory snack would hit the spot. For a real treat, cook up four or five slices of uncured bacon, chop it up finely, and roll the fat bombs in the bacon bits before freezing them. The bacon will add protein and a little fat to the macros.

1 ripe avocado, peeled
⅓ cup cocoa butter
1 tablespoon freshly squeezed lime juice

1 teaspoon chopped fresh cilantro
1 teaspoon minced jalapeño pepper
1 teaspoon minced garlic

1. Place the avocado, cocoa butter, lime juice, cilantro, jalapeño, and garlic in a blender and pulse until smooth.
2. Transfer the mixture to a bowl and place in the refrigerator until firm enough to roll into balls, about 1 hour.
3. Roll into 10 balls and place in the freezer to firm up, about 3 hours.
4. Serve frozen. Store in the freezer for up to 1 month in a sealed container.

Nutrition Tip: Avocados are high in beta-carotene and lutein, as well as folate, omega-3 fatty acids, potassium, and vitamin K. Avocados are the perfect keto food, with a 4:1 ketogenic ratio! (4 grams fat: 1 gram (protein + carb)

Per Serving
Macronutrients: Fat: 96 percent; Protein: 2 percent; Carbs: 2 percent
Ketogenic Ratio: 7:1
Calories: 94; Total Fat: 10g; Total Carbohydrates: 2g; Fiber: 1g;
Net Carbs: 1g; Protein: 0.4g; Sugar Alcohols: 0g

Creamy Tiramisu Fat Bomb

MAKES 12 / PREP TIME: 15 MINUTES, PLUS TIME TO CHILL

Tiramisu is a delectable traditional Italian dessert whose flavor profile is mimicked here in these fat bombs. Their texture can be slightly softer because of the velvety mascarpone, so make sure you chill them thoroughly. Choose the best-quality cacao possible because the taste will be superior. You can even find single-plantation chocolate powder if you have a nice organic section in your local store. Similar to wine, the taste of this powder can be affected by what grows around the beans, so try a few to find your favorite product.

½ cup cream cheese
½ cup mascarpone cheese
¼ cup cocoa butter
¼ cup almond flour

1 tablespoon cacao powder
1 tablespoon Swerve
½ teaspoon liquid coffee extract
½ cup almond meal

1. Place the cream cheese, mascarpone, cocoa butter, almond flour, cacao powder, Swerve, and coffee extract in a blender and pulse until very well mixed and smooth.
2. Scoop the mixture into balls, 2 tablespoons each, and place them on a baking sheet.
3. Freeze the balls until firm, about 1 hour.
4. Roll the balls in the almond meal and place them in a container and cover.
5. Serve frozen. Store in the freezer for up to 1 month in a sealed container.

Substitution Tip: If caffeine is not a migraine trigger for you, use a teaspoon of instant coffee instead of the extract to increase the flavor.

Per Serving
Macronutrients: Fat: 87 percent; Protein: 5 percent; Carbs: 8 percent
Ketogenic Ratio: 5:1
Calories: 156; Total Fat: 15g; Total Carbohydrates: 2g; Fiber: 1g;
Net Carbs: 1g; Protein: 2g; Sugar Alcohols: 1g

Cinnamon Coconut Fat Bomb

MAKES 12 / PREP TIME: 10 MINUTES, PLUS TIME TO CHILL

Two types of coconut—oil and shredded—are used in these scrumptious bombs, but the taste is not overpowering because of the addition of creamy almond butter and warming cinnamon. Coconut contains saturated fat but is mostly made up of medium-chain triglycerides, which are processed into ketones very efficiently and are great on a ketogenic diet.

½ cup cocoa butter
½ cup coconut oil
½ cup finely shredded unsweetened coconut

2 tablespoons almond butter
2 tablespoons Swerve
¾ teaspoon ground cinnamon

1. Place the cocoa butter, coconut oil, coconut, almond butter, Swerve, and cinnamon in a blender and pulse until very well combined.
2. Spoon the mixture into an ice cube tray, pressing it in firmly.
3. Freeze the fat bombs until very firm, 2 to 3 hours.
4. Pop the fat bombs out of the tray and place them in a container.
5. Serve frozen. Store in a sealed container for up to 1 month.

Make It Easy: Try pressing the fat bomb mixture into molds used for making chocolates, rather than ice cube trays, to create pretty guest-friendly treats. You can find these molds in most kitchen stores and craft stores.

Per Serving
Macronutrients: Fat: 98 percent; Protein: 1 percent; Carbs: 1 percent
Ketogenic Ratio: 11:1
Calories: 198; Total Fat: 22g; Total Carbohydrates: 2g; Fiber: 1g;
Net Carbs: 1g; Protein: 1g; Sugar Alcohols: 2g

Simple Cauliflower Rice

SERVES 4 / PREP TIME: 10 MINUTES / COOK TIME: 8 MINUTES

Cauliflower rice is a staple in keto cooking because it provides bulk to recipes, is low in carbs, and tastes amazing in all the dishes where you would ordinarily use a grain. Cauliflower has a mild flavor and soaks up any seasonings or spices you throw in with it. So adding cumin, coriander, cinnamon, chili powder, basil, and thyme is encouraged to enhance the dish.

1 small head cauliflower
4 tablespoons olive oil or butter

Sea salt
Freshly ground black pepper

1. Use the large holes on a box grater to rice the cauliflower into a large bowl.
2. Heat the olive oil or butter in a large skillet over medium heat.
3. Sauté the cauliflower rice until tender, stirring constantly, 6 to 8 minutes.
4. Season with salt and pepper and serve.

Make It Easy: You can purchase riced cauliflower in most stores in the salad section. Grating cauliflower can create a huge mess, so you can also use a food processor and pulse the vegetable until it is the texture you want.

Per Serving
Macronutrients: Fat: 92 percent; Protein: 3 percent; Carbs: 5 percent
Ketogenic Ratio: 7:1
Calories: 137; Total Fat: 14g; Total Carbohydrates: 3g; Fiber: 2g;
Net Carbs: 1g; Protein: 1g; Sugar Alcohols: 0g

Lemon Garlic Broccoli

SERVES 4 / PREP TIME: 10 MINUTES / COOK TIME: 11 MINUTES

Broccoli is a robust vegetable that holds up very well to sautéing, and the tightly packed floret heads soak up the buttery lemon garlic sauce. This is not a dish that can sit too long after it's completed, so make it last and place it right on the table. If you wait too long, the broccoli florets will get soggy and start to break down. This can also be made with cauliflower in the same amount.

⅓ cup butter
2 teaspoons minced garlic
2 small heads broccoli, cut into florets

Juice and zest of 1 lemon
Sea salt

1. Melt the butter in a large skillet over medium-high heat.
2. Sauté the garlic until softened, about 3 minutes.
3. Add the broccoli to the skillet and sauté until tender-crisp, stirring frequently, about 8 minutes.
4. Remove from the heat and stir in the lemon juice and lemon zest.
5. Season with salt and serve immediately.

Nutrition Tip: Garlic has been used for centuries to heal the body. This allium contains trace amounts of vitamins A, B6, and C, and iron and potassium, as well as numerous antioxidants.

Per Serving
Macronutrients: Fat: 84 percent; Protein: 7 percent; Carbs: 9 percent
Ketogenic Ratio: 2.5:1
Calories: 161; Total Fat: 15g; Total Carbohydrates: 5g; Fiber: 2g;
Net Carbs: 3g; Protein: 3g; Sugar Alcohols: 0g

Cheesy Mashed Cauliflower

SERVES 4 / PREP TIME: 10 MINUTES / COOK TIME: 30 MINUTES

Mashed cauliflower is a magical dish—velvety-textured, lush, and delicious. It holds its own against traditional high-carb mashed potatoes. You can serve your mashed cauliflower right after purée-ing instead of baking the casserole, but baking in the oven creates a tempting golden crust. You can also sprinkle shredded cheese on top of the casserole for an extra cheesy layer.

1 small head cauliflower, cut into florets
8 ounces cream cheese, cut into
   1-inch chunks
¼ cup heavy (whipping) cream

1 teaspoon minced garlic
¼ teaspoon ground nutmeg
Sea salt

1. Preheat the oven to 350°F.
2. Place a large saucepan filled with water over high heat and bring the water to a boil.
3. Blanch the cauliflower until tender, 8 to 10 minutes.
4. Drain and transfer the cauliflower to a food processor. Add the cream cheese, cream, garlic, and nutmeg. Pulse until very smooth and fluffy. Season with salt.
5. Transfer to a 9-by-9-inch casserole dish and bake until heated through and golden, about 20 minutes.
6. Serve hot.

Substitution Tip: Cream cheese is a very mild cheese that is not aged, so it's great for a migraine diet. You can also use ricotta, which is higher in calcium, and cottage cheese, but you will have to add extra butter, about 3 tablespoons, to make up the lost fat.

Per Serving
Macronutrients: Fat: 85 percent; Protein: 9 percent; Carbs: 6 percent
Ketogenic Ratio: 2.3:1
Calories: 264; Total Fat: 25g; Total Carbohydrates: 7g; Fiber: 2g;
Net Carbs: 5g; Protein: 6g; Sugar Alcohols: 0g

Asparagus with Butter and Chopped Egg

SERVES 4 / PREP TIME: 10 MINUTES / COOK TIME: 3 MINUTES

If you like hollandaise sauce, this simplified egg and butter topping will remind you of the flavor, with none of the whisking and work. Butter is made by separating the cream from milk, then churning the cream until the milk fat clumps together into a solid mass, leaving the liquid (buttermilk) behind. Butter is, of course, high in fat, about 80 percent in total or 11 grams of fat per tablespoon.

1 bunch asparagus (about 16 spears), woody ends removed

4 hardboiled eggs, chopped

⅓ cup butter, melted

Freshly ground black pepper

1. Place a large saucepan filled with water over high heat and bring to a boil.
2. Blanch the asparagus until tender-crisp, about 2 minutes.
3. Drain and arrange the asparagus on a plate. Top with the egg and drizzle with the melted butter.
4. Season with pepper and serve.

Nutrition Tip: Including vitamin B2 (riboflavin) in your diet can produce a 50 percent decrease in migraine incidence in some people. Asparagus is a good source of this nutrient.

Per Serving
Macronutrients: Fat: 83 percent; Protein: 14 percent; Carbs: 3 percent
Ketogenic Ratio: 1.9:1
Calories: 227; Total Fat: 21g; Total Carbohydrates: 4g; Fiber: 1g;
Net Carbs: 3g; Protein: 8g; Sugar Alcohols: 0g

Sesame Kale

SERVES 4 / PREP TIME: 5 MINUTES / COOK TIME: 7 MINUTES

Sesame and kale are a natural pairing. Both are strongly flavored, and the slight bitterness of the greens is offset by the richness of the sesame oil. This dish has a decidedly Asian flair with the soy sauce, scallion, and sesame, which are all common ingredients in Asian cuisine. You could add chopped bok choy and sliced red bell pepper to create a pretty stir-fry with lots of antioxidants and nutrients.

2 tablespoons sesame oil
1 pound chopped kale
1 tablespoon soy sauce

1 scallion, green and white parts, thinly sliced on a bias
2 tablespoons sesame seeds

1. Heat the oil in a large skillet over medium-high heat.
2. Sauté the kale until tender, stirring frequently, 6 to 7 minutes.
3. Remove from the heat and stir in the soy sauce.
4. Serve topped with scallion and sesame seeds.

Nutrition Tip: Kale is a deep-hued, nutrient-packed green that's exceptionally high in vitamins A, B, and C, as well as calcium, potassium, iron, magnesium, and chlorophyll.

Per Serving
Macronutrients: Fat: 74 percent; Protein: 10 percent; Carbs: 16 percent
Ketogenic Ratio: 1.3:1
Calories: 121; Total Fat: 10g; Total Carbohydrates: 8g; Fiber: 3g;
Net Carbs: 5g; Protein: 3g; Sugar Alcohols: 0g

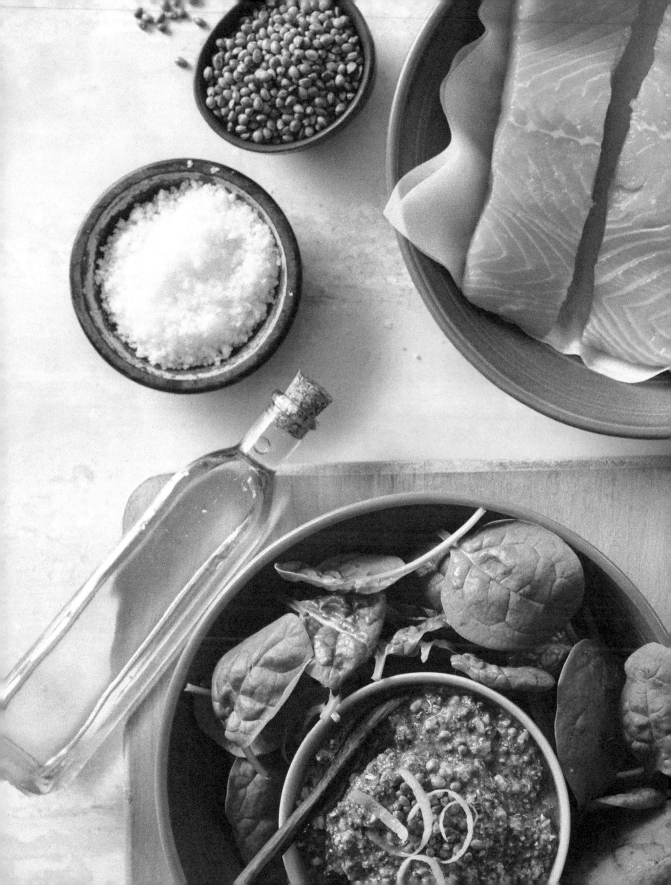

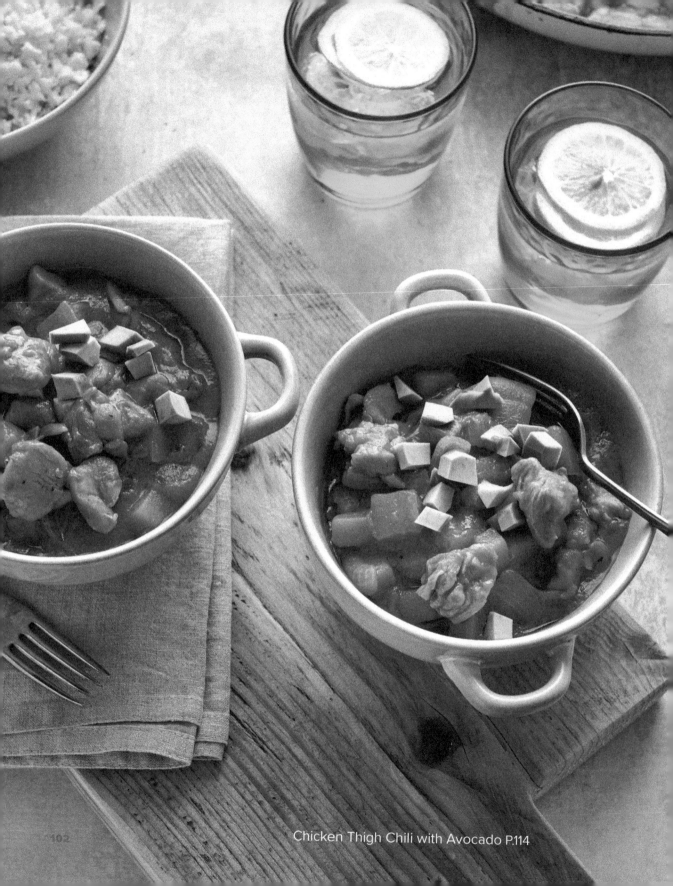

Chicken Thigh Chili with Avocado P.114

CHAPTER 7

Stews and Chilis

. . . .

Chicken Paprikash

SERVES 4 / PREP TIME: 15 MINUTES / COOK TIME: 30 MINUTES

Paprikash takes its name from the predominant spice in this flavorful stew—paprika. This Hungarian dish can be eaten as a stew or served over Simple Cauliflower Rice (page 96).

¼ cup olive oil, divided

¾ pound boneless, skinless chicken breasts, cut into ½-inch strips

1 medium onion, sliced

1 red bell pepper, diced

1 tablespoon minced garlic

½ cup low-sodium chicken stock or Chicken Bone Broth (page 207)

½ cup canned coconut milk

¼ cup no-salt-added tomato paste

3 tablespoons smoked paprika

½ cup sour cream

Sea salt

Freshly ground black pepper

2 tablespoons chopped fresh parsley

1. Heat 2 tablespoons of olive oil in a large skillet over medium-high heat.
2. Brown the chicken until cooked through, about 10 minutes, and transfer to a plate using a slotted spoon.
3. Add the remaining olive oil and sauté the onion, bell pepper, and garlic until softened, about 4 minutes.
4. Stir in the reserved cooked chicken, chicken stock, coconut milk, tomato paste, and paprika.
5. Cover the skillet and simmer, stirring occasionally, until the chicken and vegetables are very tender, about 15 minutes.
6. Stir in the sour cream and simmer an additional 1 minute.
7. Season with salt and pepper and serve topped with parsley.

Per Serving

Macronutrients: Fat: 67 percent; Protein: 22 percent; Carbs: 11 percent

Ketogenic Ratio: 0.9:1

Calories: 378; Total Fat: 28g; Total Carbohydrates: 14g; Fiber: 4g; Net Carbs: 10g; Protein: 21g; Sugar Alcohols: 0g

Seafood Coconut Stew

SERVES 4 / PREP TIME: 15 MINUTES / PREP TIME: 30 MINUTES

In the past, stews were often made to use up extra fish, shrimp, or scallops, so don't think you have to stick with whole salmon fillets in this dish. You can also throw in frozen seafood if you add about 10 minutes to the cooking time. Yellow bell pepper adds a lovely, festive color to this recipe, as well as a hefty quantity of vitamin C—more than other bell peppers. Yellow bell peppers contain over 75 percent of your daily requirement in this serving size.

¼ cup olive oil

1 onion, chopped

1 yellow bell pepper, chopped

1 cup sliced mushrooms

1 tablespoon minced garlic

2 teaspoons peeled, grated fresh ginger

2 cups low-sodium chicken stock or Chicken Bone Broth (page 207)

1 cup canned coconut milk

2 teaspoons ground turmeric

½ pound salmon fillets, diced

½ pound shrimp, peeled, deveined, and each cut into 4 pieces

1 cup cauliflower florets

Sea salt

Freshly ground black pepper

1 cup shredded kale

1. Heat the olive oil in a large stockpot over medium-high heat.
2. Sauté the onion, bell pepper, mushrooms, garlic, and ginger until the vegetables are softened, about 5 minutes.
3. Add the chicken stock, coconut milk, and turmeric and bring the soup to a boil.
4. Add the fish, shrimp, and cauliflower and reduce the heat to low. Simmer the soup until the fish is cooked through, about 5 minutes.

Continued on next page

5. Season with salt and pepper.
6. Stir in the kale and simmer 4 more minutes. Serve immediately.

. . . .

Substitution Tip: Shellfish allergies are one of the most serious, so eliminate the shrimp if you have this issue. Double up on the fish or add another type of fish, such as haddock or halibut, for a different taste and texture.

Per Serving
Macronutrients: Fat: 68 percent; Protein: 23 percent; Carbs: 9 percent
Ketogenic Ratio: 0.9:1
Calories: 426; Total Fat: 32g; Total Carbohydrates: 12g; Fiber: 3g;
Net Carbs: 9g; Protein: 25g; Sugar Alcohols: 0g

Moroccan Almond Stew

SERVES 4 / PREP TIME: 15 MINUTES / COOK TIME: 25 MINUTES

Moroccan food is complex, gloriously hued, and created with ingredients that you probably already have on hand in your refrigerator and pantry—vegetables, aromatics like onion and garlic, spices, almond butter, and tofu. This meal could easily include meat like lamb or chicken if you want to increase the protein. If you do add protein, use only 8 ounces and add 4 to 6 tablespoons of oil to balance the ratio. Just sauté the chopped meat in the coconut oil until cooked through and follow the instructions through to the end.

¼ cup coconut oil, divided

14 ounces extra-firm tofu, diced

1 onion, chopped

1 red bell pepper, diced

2 celery stalks, chopped

1 tablespoon minced garlic

1 jalapeño pepper, finely diced

2 cups small cauliflower florets

2 cups low-sodium vegetable stock

½ cup canned coconut milk

2 tablespoons curry paste (hot or mild, to taste)

1 teaspoon ground cumin

Juice of 1 lime

¼ cup almond butter

¼ cup hemp hearts

2 tablespoons chopped fresh cilantro

1. Heat 2 tablespoons of oil in a large pot over medium-high heat.
2. Sauté the tofu until crispy and lightly browned, about 5 minutes. Transfer to a plate using a slotted spoon.
3. Add the remaining oil and sauté the onion, bell pepper, celery, garlic, and jalapeño until softened, about 5 minutes.

Continued on next page

4. Add the tofu back to the pot along with the cauliflower, stock, coconut milk, curry paste, and cumin. Bring to a boil.
5. Reduce the heat to low and simmer until the vegetables are tender, about 10 minutes.
6. Stir in the lime juice, almond butter, hemp hearts, and cilantro, and simmer 2 minutes more. Serve.

. . . .

Substitution Tip: A more traditional preparation of this dish uses peanut butter instead of almond butter. If you prefer it, swap the nut butters and top the stew with some chopped peanuts for a crunchy texture.

Per Serving
Macronutrients: Fat: 71 percent; Protein: 16 percent; Carbs: 13 percent
Ketogenic Ratio: 1.2:1
Calories: 470; Total Fat: 37g; Total Carbohydrates: 20g; Fiber: 7g;
Net Carbs: 13g; Protein: 19g; Sugar Alcohols: 0g

Savory Lamb Stew

SERVES 4 / PREP TIME: 20 MINUTES / COOK TIME: 35 MINUTES

Lamb stew is a popular dish in North Africa and Ireland, although the main ingredient in Ireland would be mutton instead of lamb. Sheep were kept until old age to use the valuable wool and milk. The lamb in this version is ground instead of chunks to cut down on the cooking time.

¼ cup olive oil
1 pound ground lamb
1 onion, chopped
2 cups halved mushrooms
1 tablespoon minced garlic
1 teaspoon peeled, grated fresh ginger
½ teaspoon ground turmeric
½ teaspoon ground cinnamon

¼ teaspoon ground cloves
2 cups diced raw or frozen pumpkin
2 cups low-sodium beef stock or Beef Bone Broth (page 208)
1 tablespoon chopped fresh thyme
Sea salt
Freshly ground black pepper

1. Heat the olive oil in a large stockpot on medium-high heat.
2. Brown the lamb until cooked through, stirring occasionally, about 10 minutes.
3. Add the onion, mushrooms, garlic, ginger, turmeric, cinnamon, and cloves. Sauté until the vegetables are softened, about 5 minutes.
4. Stir in the pumpkin, beef stock, and thyme and bring the stew to a boil.
5. Reduce the heat to low and simmer until the pumpkin is tender, about 20 minutes.
6. Season with salt and pepper and serve.

Per Serving
Macronutrients: Fat: 74 percent; Protein: 19 percent; Carbs: 7 percent
Ketogenic Ratio: 1.3:1
Calories: 489; Total Fat: 40g; Total Carbohydrates: 9g; Fiber: 2g;
Net Carbs: 7g; Protein: 23g; Sugar Alcohols: 0g

Beef Stroganoff

SERVES 4 / PREP TIME: 15 MINUTES / COOK TIME: 40 MINUTES

Stroganoff is a Russian dish consisting of tender beef strips in a rich, creamy mushroom sauce. Sour cream is often a welcome addition to the recipe, but this version is dairy-free. Rib eye steak is a good choice as the base because it is high in fat and very tender. This cut is generously marbled. Like all keto meals, the high fat content of rib eye will help you feel full longer.

3 tablespoons olive oil

1 pound rib eye steak, cut into thin strips

1 onion, chopped

2 cups sliced button mushrooms

1 tablespoon minced garlic

1 cup low-sodium beef broth or Beef Bone Broth (page 208)

1 cup canned coconut milk

Sea salt

Freshly ground black pepper

2 tablespoons chopped fresh parsley

1. Heat the olive oil in a large skillet over medium-high heat.
2. Sauté the beef strips until they are lightly browned, about 10 minutes. Remove the beef from the skillet using a slotted spoon and set aside on a plate.
3. Add the onion, mushrooms, and garlic to the skillet and sauté until tender, about 8 minutes.

4. Stir in the beef broth and coconut milk.
5. Add the beef and any accumulated juices back into the skillet and simmer the stroganoff until the beef is very tender, about 20 minutes.
6. Season with salt and pepper. Serve garnished with chopped parsley.

. . . .

Make It Easy: This recipe can be made in a slow cooker, with stellar results. Brown the beef and add it with the remaining ingredients, except for the parsley, to a slow cooker. Cook on low heat for 8 hours. Serve topped with parsley.

Per Serving
Macronutrients: Fat: 77 percent; Protein: 18 percent; Carbs: 5 percent
Ketogenic Ratio: 1.6:1
Calories: 512; Total Fat: 44g; Total Carbohydrates: 6g; Fiber: 1g;
Net Carbs: 5g; Protein: 23g; Sugar Alcohols: 0g

White Chili

White chili usually refers to chili that uses chicken instead of beef, but this recipe also adds cauliflower and coconut milk, to make it truly white. Although the origins of chili are a little vague, the green, white, and red color palate of this dish pays tribute to possible Mexican roots. Ground cumin adds a lemony complexity to the chili.

¼ cup coconut oil, divided

1 pound boneless, skinless chicken breasts, diced

1 onion, diced

1 red bell pepper, diced

1 green bell pepper, diced

1 tablespoon minced garlic

3 cups small cauliflower florets

2 cups canned coconut milk

2 tablespoons chili powder

1 teaspoon ground cumin

Pinch red pepper flakes

¼ cup chopped fresh cilantro

1. Heat 2 tablespoons of oil in a large saucepan over medium-high heat.
2. Sauté the chicken until just cooked through, 10 to 12 minutes. Transfer the chicken to a plate using a slotted spoon.
3. Add the remaining oil and sauté the onion, red and green bell peppers, and garlic until softened, about 5 minutes.

4. Stir in the cooked chicken, cauliflower, coconut milk, chili powder, cumin, and red pepper flakes.
5. Bring the chili to a boil, then reduce the heat to low and simmer until the chicken and vegetables are tender, about 20 minutes.
6. Serve topped with cilantro.

. . . .

Make It Easy: This recipe is simple but takes a little time to create, especially if your schedule is packed. To save time, use leftover cooked chicken from dinner the night before, instead of sautéing raw poultry.

Per Serving
Macronutrients: Fat: 70 percent; Protein: 22 percent; Carbs: 8 percent
Ketogenic Ratio: 1.1
Calories: 401; Total Fat: 31g; Total Carbohydrates: 13g; Fiber: 4g;
Net Carbs: 9g; Protein: 22g; Sugar Alcohols: 0g

Chicken Thigh Chili with Avocado

SERVES 4 / PREP TIME: 15 MINUTES / COOK TIME: 40 MINUTES

Chicken thighs are a juicy, flavorful cut of poultry—more flavorful than the favored chicken breast and less expensive, as well. This is a pretty, slightly sweet chili that would be wonderful spooned over cauliflower rice or even into a cold lettuce wrap.

3 tablespoons olive oil, divided

1 pound boneless, skinless chicken thighs, diced

1 onion, chopped

2 jalapeño peppers, minced

1 tablespoon minced garlic

2 cups diced raw or frozen pumpkin

1 cup low-sodium chicken stock or Chicken Bone Broth (page 207)

1 cup canned coconut milk

3 tablespoons no-salt-added tomato paste

3 tablespoons chili powder

Juice of 1 lime

1 avocado, diced

1. Heat 2 tablespoons of olive oil in a large saucepan over medium-high heat.
2. Sauté the chicken until just cooked through, 10 to 12 minutes. Transfer the chicken to a plate using a slotted spoon.
3. Add the remaining olive oil and sauté the onion, jalapeños, and garlic until softened, about 5 minutes.

4. Stir in the cooked chicken, pumpkin, chicken stock, coconut milk, tomato paste, chili powder, and lime juice.
5. Bring the chili to a boil, then reduce the heat to low and simmer until the chicken and vegetables are tender, about 20 minutes.
6. Serve topped with avocado.

Nutrition Tip: Pumpkins are extremely rich in beta-carotene and vitamins B, C, D, and E, as well as iron, potassium, and copper. This fruit supports a healthy digestive system and boosts immunity.

Per Serving
Macronutrients: Fat: 70 percent; Protein: 17 percent; Carbs: 13 percent
Ketogenic Ratio: 1.2:1
Calories: 461; Total Fat: 36g; Total Carbohydrates: 18g; Fiber: 7g;
Net Carbs: 11g; Protein: 20g; Sugar Alcohols: 0g

Ground Lamb Chili

SERVES 4 / PREP TIME: 15 MINUTES / COOK TIME: 45 MINUTES

Lamb has an assertive flavor that can stand up to and blend
beautifully with strong chili powder. This means if you like heat,
you can experiment with different types of chili powder,
from searing hot to mild almost sweet.

¼ cup olive oil

1 pound ground lamb

1 onion, chopped

½ fennel bulb, diced

1 red bell pepper, chopped

1 tablespoon minced garlic

3 tablespoons chili powder

1 teaspoon ground cumin

1 teaspoon ground coriander

¼ teaspoon red pepper flakes

2 cups low-sodium chicken stock or
    Chicken Bone Broth (page 207)

1 cup canned coconut milk

2 tablespoons chopped fresh cilantro

1. Heat the olive oil in a large stockpot over medium-high heat.
2. Sauté the lamb until it is cooked through, about 15 minutes.
3. Add the onion, fennel, bell pepper, and garlic and sauté until softened, about 6 minutes.
4. Stir in the chili powder, cumin, coriander, and red pepper flakes and sauté 4 minutes.
5. Stir in the chicken stock and coconut milk and bring the mixture to a boil.
6. Simmer until the vegetables are tender and the flavors have mellowed, about 20 minutes.
7. Serve topped with cilantro.

Per Serving

Macronutrients: Fat: 78 percent; Protein: 15 percent; Carbs: 7 percent

Ketogenic Ratio: 1.6:1

Calories: 600; Total Fat: 52g; Total Carbohydrates: 12g; Fiber: 4g;
Net Carbs: 8g; Protein: 22g; Sugar Alcohols: 0g

Classic Beef Chili

SERVES 6 / PREP TIME: 15 MINUTES / COOK TIME: 1 HOUR AND 30 MINUTES

When you think of a basic chili—ground beef, peppers, onions, and a nicely spiced tomato-based sauce—you are probably thinking of something close to this recipe. The one slightly different ingredient is ancho chili powder. It's made from a milder dried pepper, poblano, and lands low on the Scoville heat scale at 1,000 to 1,500. Regular chili powder is made of dried jalapeño peppers and is about 2,500 heat units. So even those who don't like spicy food will enjoy this tasty meal.

¼ cup olive oil

1 pound ground beef

1 onion, chopped

1 green bell pepper, chopped

1 tablespoon minced garlic

3 tablespoons ancho chili powder

2 teaspoons ground cumin

1 teaspoon ground coriander

1 teaspoon smoked paprika

2 cups low-sodium beef stock or Beef Bone Broth (page 208)

½ cup no-salt-added tomato paste

1 cup sour cream

1. Heat the olive oil in a large stockpot over medium-high heat.
2. Sauté the beef until it is cooked through, about 15 minutes.
3. Add the onion, bell pepper, and garlic and sauté until softened, about 6 minutes.
4. Stir in the chili powder, cumin, coriander, and paprika and sauté 4 minutes.
5. Stir in the beef stock and tomato paste and bring the mixture to a boil.

Continued on next page

6. Simmer until the sauce thickens and the flavors have mellowed, about 1 hour.
7. Serve topped with 2½ tablespoons sour cream.

- -

Substitution Tip: If you have an issue with dairy, swap the sour cream for a good-quality vegan sour cream or plain coconut yogurt in the same amount. This will drop the fat percentage, so top with diced avocado and add another 2 to 3 tablespoons of olive oil to the recipe to keep the ratio intact.

Per Serving

Macronutrients: Fat: 70 percent; Protein: 18 percent; Carbs: 12 percent

Ketogenic Ratio: 1.1:1

Calories: 410; Total Fat: 32g; Total Carbohydrates: 14g; Fiber: 3g;
Net Carbs: 11g; Protein: 18g; Sugar Alcohols: 0g

Texas Style Beef Chili

SERVES 6 / PREP TIME: 20 MINUTES / COOK TIME: 1 HOUR AND 45 MINUTES

This is an authentic chili con carne with chunks of beef, complex spices, heat, and the unexpected richness of cocoa to lift the dish to another flavor level. If you do not have an issue with coffee, you can swap out 2 cups of beef broth for 2 cups of brewed coffee. Coffee adds earthiness and is a perfect pairing with the other ingredients.

3 tablespoons ground chipotle chili powder

2 tablespoons ground cumin

1 tablespoon dried oregano

½ teaspoon ground cinnamon

¼ cup olive oil

2 pounds beef chuck roast, cut into 1-inch cubes

1 onion, diced

2 jalapeño peppers, finely chopped

1 tablespoon minced garlic

6 cups low-sodium beef stock or Beef Bone Broth (page 208)

½ cup no-salt-added tomato paste

1 tablespoon unsweetened cocoa powder

1 cup sour cream

1. In a small bowl, mix together the chili powder, cumin, oregano, and cinnamon until well combined. Set aside.
2. Heat the olive oil in a large saucepan over medium-high heat.
3. Sauté the beef until browned, about 10 minutes, and transfer to a plate using a slotted spoon.
4. Sauté the onion, jalapeños, and garlic until softened, about 4 minutes.
5. Add the beef back to the pot, along with any accumulated juices on the plate, and the spice mixture. Stir to evenly coat.

Continued on next page

6. Stir in the beef stock, tomato paste, and cocoa powder.
7. Bring the chili to a boil, cover, and reduce the heat to low. Simmer until the sauce is thickened and the beef is very tender, stirring occasionally, about 1½ hours.
8. Serve topped with sour cream.

Per Serving

Macronutrients: Fat: 72 percent; Protein: 20 percent; Carbs: 8 percent

Ketogenic Ratio: 1.17:1

Calories: ¼ cup tomato paste: Total Fat: 0g; Protein: 1g; Total Carbs: 1g; Fiber: 0g; Net Carbs: 1g
1 ½ cups sour cream: Total Fat: 11g; Protein: 1g; Total Carbs: 2g; Fiber: 0g; Net Carbs: 2g
1 avocado, diced: Total Fat: 4g; Protein: 0g; Total Carbs: 2g; Fiber: 2g; Net Carbs: 0g
Total Calories: 683; Total Fat: 55g; Protein: 35g; Total Carbs: 12g; Fiber: 4g; Net Carbs: 8g

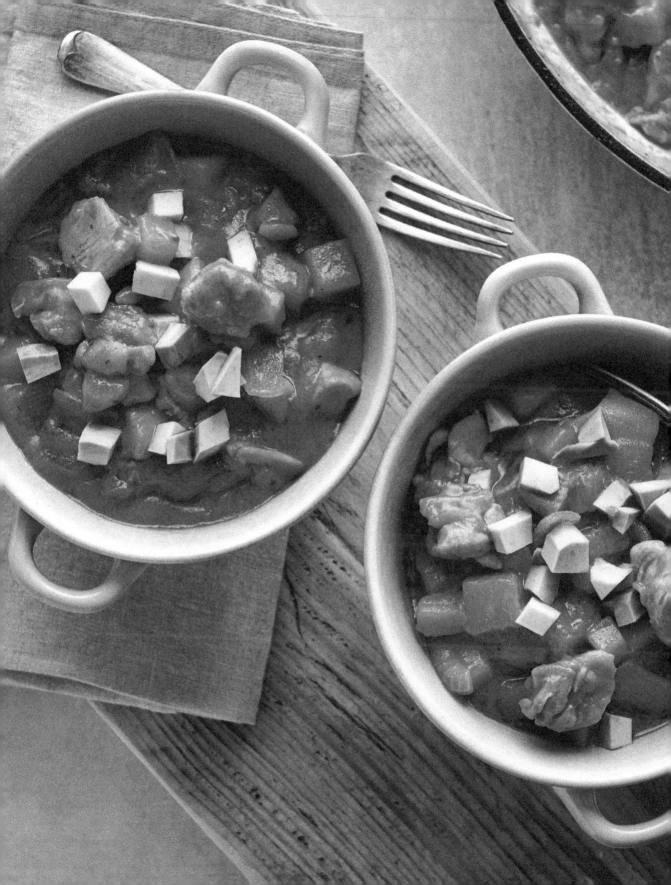

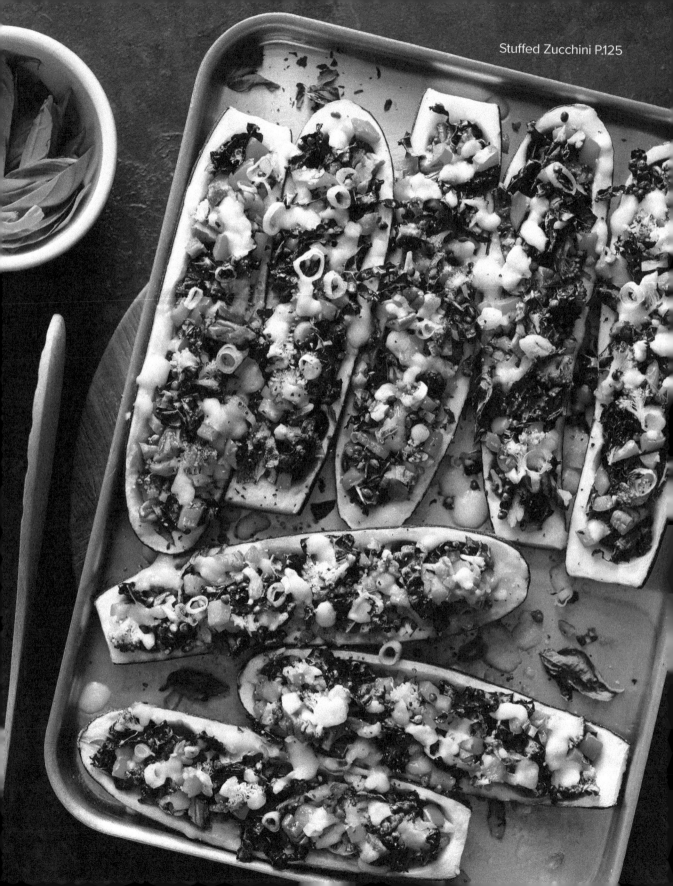

Stuffed Zucchini P.125

CHAPTER 8

Meatless Mains

. . . .

Ginger Vegetable Tofu Scramble

SERVES 4 / PREP TIME: 15 MINUTES / COOK TIME: 19 MINUTES

Scrambled tofu is very similar to scrambled eggs in texture and has the added benefit of soaking up all the flavor of the surrounding ingredients, such as the ginger in this recipe. Fresh ginger is different than the dried, ground product you find on the spice rack. Fresh is less intensely flavored but contains more gingerol and other powerful healing compounds, which can help block prostaglandins, an inflammatory substance. Ginger can also help reduce any migraine-related nausea.

¼ cup coconut oil

½ cup chopped onion

2 teaspoons minced garlic

2 teaspoons peeled, grated fresh ginger

14 ounces extra-firm tofu, pressed, drained, and diced

2 teaspoons garam masala

2 cups shredded kale

1 cup sliced baby bok choy

1. Melt the coconut oil in a large skillet over medium-high heat.
2. Sauté the onion, garlic, and ginger until softened, about 3 minutes.
3. Add the tofu and sauté, breaking it up into chunks, about 10 minutes.
4. Stir in the garam masala and sauté 1 minute.
5. Add the kale and bok choy and sauté until the greens are wilted, about 5 minutes.

Nutrition Tip: Bok choy is a wonderful addition to a healthy diet because it is a good source of vitamins A, C, and K. It also boosts the immune system and promotes healthy brain function.

Per Serving

Macronutrients: Fat: 70 percent; Protein: 20 percent; Carbs: 10 percent

Ketogenic Ratio: 1:1

Calories: 245; Total Fat: 19g; Total Carbohydrates: 11g; Fiber: 3g; Net Carbs: 8g; Protein: 12g; Sugar Alcohols: 0g

Stuffed Zucchini

SERVES 4 / PREP TIME: 20 MINUTES / COOK TIME: 30 MINUTES

Stuffed vegetables are a staple of vegetarian cuisine because they are fun to create and have the benefit of heaping many nutritious ingredients in a handy edible container. Brassica vegetables, dark leafy greens, nuts, and protein-packed hemp hearts form the substance of this hearty filling.

3 tablespoons olive oil

1 cup finely chopped broccoli

1 red bell pepper, chopped

1 cup shredded kale

1 scallion, white and green parts, chopped

½ cup finely chopped pecans

¼ cup hemp hearts

1 tablespoon chopped fresh basil

Sea salt

Freshly ground black pepper

4 medium zucchini

1 cup crumbled goat cheese

1. Preheat the oven to 350°F.
2. Heat the olive oil in a large skillet over medium-high heat.
3. Sauté the broccoli, bell pepper, kale, and scallion until tender, 6 to 8 minutes.
4. Stir in the pecans, hemp hearts, and basil.
5. Season the filling with salt and pepper.
6. Cut a thin, lengthwise layer off the zucchini and scoop out the insides of the vegetables, leaving the outer shell intact. (Save the zucchini flesh for another meal.)
7. Spoon the filling into the zucchini shells and top with goat cheese.
8. Bake until the filling is warmed through and the cheese is melted, about 20 minutes.

Per Serving

Macronutrients: Fat: 77 percent; Protein: 15 percent; Carbs: 8 percent

Ketogenic Ratio: 1.5:1

Calories: 408; Total Fat: 35g; Total Carbohydrates: 16g; Fiber: 7g;

Net Carbs: 9g; Protein: 15g; Sugar Alcohols: 0g

Almond Fried Goat Cheese

SERVES 6 / PREP TIME: 20 MINUTES, PLUS TIME TO CHILL / COOK TIME: 10 MINUTES

Breaking through the golden nut layer of these patties to the creamy cheese interior with the side of your fork is a sublime culinary experience. The melt-in-your-mouth texture of the rich cheese, accented by crunchy bits of sweet fried almond, is exceptional, especially when served with a lovely, fresh mixed green salad.

1 (16-ounce) goat cheese log
1½ cups almond meal, divided
2 eggs, beaten
1 tablespoon chopped fresh parsley

¼ teaspoon sea salt
¼ teaspoon freshly ground black pepper
½ cup avocado oil

1. Place the goat cheese log in the freezer for 30 minutes to firm it up.
2. Add ½ cup of almond meal to a small bowl.
3. Add the eggs to a second bowl.
4. Place the remaining almond meal, parsley, salt, and pepper in a third bowl, stirring to combine.
5. Slice the goat cheese into ½-inch-thick slices using dental floss or fishing line.
6. Carefully dredge the goat cheese in the almond meal, then the eggs, and finally the almond-parsley mixture until entirely breaded.
7. Heat the oil in a large skillet over medium-high heat.
8. Fry the breaded cheese until golden brown, turning once, about 10 minutes in total.

Per Serving
Macronutrients: Fat: 82 percent; Protein: 15 percent; Carbs: 3 percent
Ketogenic Ratio: 2.2:1
Calories: 569; Total Fat: 52g; Total Carbohydrates: 4g; Fiber: 2g; Net Carbs: 2g; Protein: 22g; Sugar Alcohols: 0g

Stir-Fried Sesame Broccoli

SERVES 4 / PREP TIME: 15 MINUTES / COOK TIME: 15 MINUTES

Stir-fries are a fantastic, quick way to create a healthy meal with inexpensive ingredients. You can use any vegetable, but the combination of dark green broccoli, red peppers, and yellow zucchini is pretty on the plate. Serve over cauliflower rice to bulk up the meal, or as a hearty side dish with a nice fish fillet. Yellow zucchini can be confused with yellow summer squash, but it is okay to use either because they have similar taste and nutrition profiles. Both contain heart-healthy potassium, antioxidants, and vitamin C.

¼ cup sesame oil

1 tablespoon peeled, grated fresh ginger

2 teaspoons minced garlic

3 cups broccoli florets

1 red bell pepper, cut into thin strips

1 yellow zucchini, sliced

1 scallion, white and green parts, thinly sliced

1 tablespoon chopped fresh cilantro

¼ cup hemp hearts

1. Heat the oil in a large skillet over medium-high heat.
2. Sauté the ginger and garlic until softened, about 3 minutes.
3. Add the broccoli, bell pepper, zucchini, and scallion and sauté until tender-crisp, about 12 minutes.
4. Stir in the cilantro and serve topped with hemp hearts.

Nutrition Tip: Broccoli is a stellar source of vitamins C and K, as well as fiber.

Per Serving

Macronutrients: Fat: 74 percent; Protein: 9 percent; Carbs: 17 percent

Ketogenic Ratio: 1.8:1

Calories: 220; Total Fat: 18g; Total Carbohydrates: 9g; Fiber: 4g; Net Carbs: 5g; Protein: 5g; Sugar Alcohols: 0g

Roasted Spaghetti Squash Casserole

SERVES 4 / PREP TIME: 25 MINUTES / COOK TIME: 1 HOUR AND 5 MINUTES

Casseroles save time in the kitchen and are often family favorites because they are a mixture of tasty ingredients in one convenient dish. Spaghetti squash is a delicious low-carb (about 8 grams net carbs per cup) option for keto dishes. It's also an excellent source of fiber, calcium, and copper, and has plenty of beta-carotene, fiber, potassium, and vitamins A, B3, B5, B6, and C.

1 small spaghetti squash, halved and seeded

3 tablespoons coconut oil, plus more for greasing the casserole dish

2 cups chopped cauliflower

2 celery stalks, chopped

1 cup shredded spinach

1 cup cream cheese

2 tablespoons nutritional yeast

1 tablespoon chopped fresh basil

Sea salt

Freshly ground black pepper

1. Preheat the oven to 400°F.
2. Rub the cut side of the spaghetti squash with the coconut oil and place the squash, cut-side down, on a baking sheet.
3. Bake the squash until it is soft, 30 to 35 minutes. Remove the squash from the oven and let it cool for 10 minutes.

4. Scoop the cooked squash strands out and transfer them to a large bowl.
5. Add the cauliflower, celery, spinach, cream cheese, nutritional yeast, and basil to the bowl and stir to combine. Season with salt and pepper.
6. Lightly grease a 9-by-9-inch casserole dish with coconut oil.
7. Spoon the squash mixture into the casserole dish and bake until warmed through and the vegetables are tender, about 30 minutes.

....

Make It Easy: Microwaving the spaghetti squash can save time. Carefully stab the squash deeply with a sharp knife several times. Set the squash cut-side down in a microwave-safe dish and add ¼ cup of water to the dish. Microwave on high for 12 to 15 minutes. Then cut the squash and scoop out the seeds. Handle with care—it will be hot!

Per Serving
Macronutrients: Fat: 76 percent; Protein: 10 percent; Carbs: 14 percent
Ketogenic Ratio: 1.5:1
Calories: 368; Total Fat: 31g; Total Carbohydrates: 18g; Fiber: 5g;
Net Carbs: 13g; Protein: 9g; Sugar Alcohols: 0g

Pumpkin Seed and Swiss Chard Stuffed Portobello Mushrooms

SERVES: 4 / PREP TIME: 10 MINUTES / COOK TIME: 35 MINUTES

Portobello mushrooms are often used in vegetarian and vegan recipes because of their meaty texture and versatility. Crunchy pumpkin stand in as the bulk of the stuffing and are very high in magnesium.

4 large Portobello mushroom caps
5 tablespoons olive oil, divided
1 cup chopped Swiss chard
½ onion, chopped
1 tablespoon minced garlic
2 teaspoons chopped fresh thyme

1½ cups pumpkin seeds
¼ cup store-bought balsamic vinaigrette
Sea salt
Freshly ground black pepper
½ cup shredded Cheddar cheese

1. Preheat the oven to 350°F.
2. Use a spoon to scoop the black gills out of the mushrooms, then massage 2 tablespoons of olive oil all over them. Place the mushrooms hollow-side up on a baking sheet.
3. Heat the remaining olive oil in a large skillet over medium-high heat.
4. Sauté the Swiss chard, onion, garlic, and thyme until the vegetables are tender, about 10 minutes.
5. Stir in the pumpkin seeds and balsamic vinaigrette and season the filling with salt and pepper.
6. Divide the filling among the mushroom caps and top with shredded Cheddar.
7. Bake until tender, about 25 minutes.

Per Serving

Macronutrients: Fat: 79 percent; Protein: 14 percent; Carbs: 7 percent
Ketogenic Ratio: 1.6:1
Calories: 517; Total Fat: 46g; Total Carbohydrates: 14g; Fiber: 4g; Net Carbs: 10g; Protein: 19g; Sugar Alcohols: 0g

Vegetable Hash

SERVES 4 / PREP TIME: 15 MINUTES / COOK TIME: 20 MINUTES

Hash is most often associated with potatoes and breakfast, but it actually is from the French *hacher*, meaning "to chop," and describes chopped vegetables and meats cooked together. This version varies in texture and has a delightful cheesy taste from the nutritional yeast. Nutritional yeast is not the same as the yeast you use to make bread—it's the same species but is inactive.

3 tablespoons avocado oil

1 onion, chopped

1 tablespoon minced garlic

4 cups chopped cauliflower

2 zucchini, diced

2 cups chopped kale

1 cup chopped pecans

2 tablespoons nutritional yeast

1 tablespoon chopped fresh oregano

Freshly ground black pepper

1 avocado, diced

1. Heat the oil in a large skillet over medium-high heat.
2. Sauté the onion and garlic until softened, about 3 minutes.
3. Add the cauliflower, zucchini, and kale and sauté until the vegetables are tender, about 15 minutes.
4. Stir in the pecans, nutritional yeast, and oregano and sauté for 2 minutes.
5. Remove from the heat and season with pepper.
6. Serve topped with avocado.

Per Serving

Macronutrients: Fat: 77 percent; Protein: 9 percent; Carbs: 14 percent

Ketogenic Ratio: 1.8:1

Calories: 456; Total Fat: 39g; Total Carbohydrates: 24g; Fiber: 12g;
Net Carbs: 12g; Protein: 10g; Sugar Alcohols: 0g

Mediterranean Spiralized Zucchini

SERVES 4 / PREP TIME: 15 MINUTES / COOK TIME: 10 MINUTES

Olives bring a flavorful briny taste to this "pasta" dish and add that Mediterranean flare. Kalamata olives can be an issue for some migraine sufferers because they can contain histamine and tyramine, but you will know if this food is a problem for you. This fruit is high in fiber, vitamin E, and iron.

3 tablespoons olive oil
1 tablespoon butter
1 tablespoon minced garlic
1 cup chopped Swiss chard
½ cup sliced Kalamata olives

2 tablespoons chopped fresh basil
3 zucchini, spiralized
Sea salt
Freshly ground black pepper
1 cup shredded fresh mozzarella cheese

1. Heat the olive oil and butter in a large skillet over medium-high heat.
2. Sauté the garlic until softened, about 2 minutes.
3. Add the Swiss chard, olives, and basil and sauté until the greens are wilted, about 8 minutes.
4. Stir in the zucchini and toss to combine.
5. Season with salt and pepper.
6. Serve topped with mozzarella cheese.

Make It Easy: Spiralized vegetables are an easy-to-find prepared ingredient in most produce sections of grocery stores, due to their popularity. Look for zucchini, summer squash, and other combinations for simple, delicious recipes.

Per Serving
Macronutrients: Fat: 80 percent; Protein: 16 percent; Carbs: 4 percent
Ketogenic Ratio: 1.4:1
Calories: 281; Total Fat: 25g; Total Carbohydrates: 10g; Fiber: 3g;
Net Carbs: 7g; Protein: 11g; Sugar Alcohols: 0g

Konjac Noodles with Spinach Hemp Pesto and Goat Cheese

SERVES 4 / PREP TIME: 15 MINUTES / COOK TIME: 10 MINUTES

Konjac noodles, garlicky pesto, mushrooms, and creamy goat cheese create a sophisticated meal with no work and very little time. Look for a harder goat cheese that crumbles better than the soft product, so it disperses more easily throughout the noodles. You could also use spiralized zucchini in this recipe.

½ cup Spinach Hemp Pesto (page 204)

2 cups sliced mushrooms

30 ounces konjac noodles, such as NuPasta, drained and rinsed

1 cup crumbled goat cheese

1. Place a large skillet over medium heat. Add the pesto and mushrooms.
2. Sauté the mushrooms until lightly caramelized, about 8 minutes.
3. Add the noodles to the skillet and toss until they are heated through, about 2 minutes.
4. Serve topped with goat cheese.

Nutrition Tip: Konjac noodles contain no fat or protein, but they are a wonderful choice for pasta dishes because they are 97 percent water and made entirely of fiber. These noodles help stabilize blood sugar and may help lower cholesterol levels.

Per Serving
Macronutrients: Fat: 67 percent; Protein: 15 percent; Carbs: 18 percent
Ketogenic Ratio: 1.3:1
Calories: 187; Total Fat: 14g; Total Carbohydrates: 10g; Fiber: 6g;
Net Carbs: 4g; Protein: 7g; Sugar Alcohols: 0g

"Fettuccini" with Avocado Alfredo

SERVES 4 / PREP TIME: 25 MINUTES / COOK TIME: 2 MINUTES

If you have a large, colorful pottery serving bowl, use it to assemble this glorious-looking recipe, which already has a festive appearance. Yellow, deep green, and creamy pale green create a meal that is spring on a plate.

2 green zucchini, cut into thin ribbons with a peeler

2 yellow zucchini, cut into thin ribbons with a peeler

1 avocado, peeled

1 cup cream cheese

½ cup heavy (whipping) cream

1 tablespoon nutritional yeast

2 teaspoons minced garlic

Freshly ground black pepper

2 tablespoons chopped fresh parsley

1. Place a medium pot of water on high heat and bring to a boil.
2. Blanch the zucchini ribbons for 2 minutes. Remove from the water using a slotted spoon and drain under cold water.
3. Pat the ribbons dry with paper towels and transfer to a large bowl.
4. Place the avocado, cream cheese, cream, nutritional yeast, and garlic in a blender and process until completely smooth. Season with pepper.
5. Add the sauce to the ribbons and toss to coat.
6. Serve topped with parsley.

Per Serving

Macronutrients: Fat: 83 percent; Protein: 9 percent; Carbs: 8 percent

Ketogenic Ratio: 2:1

Calories: 411; Total Fat: 38g; Total Carbohydrates: 15g; Fiber: 5g; Net Carbs: 10g; Protein: 9g; Sugar Alcohols: 0g

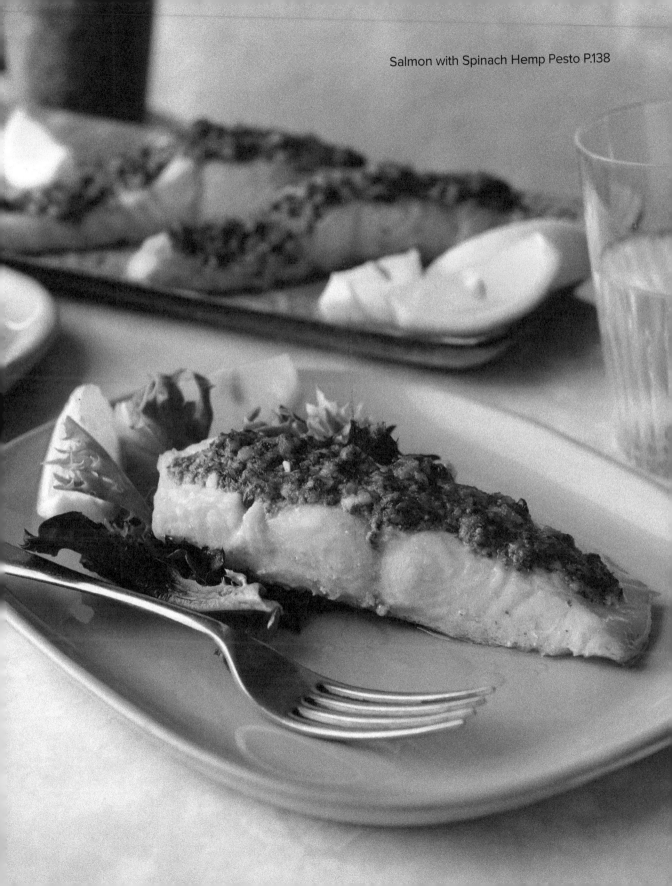

Salmon with Spinach Hemp Pesto P.138

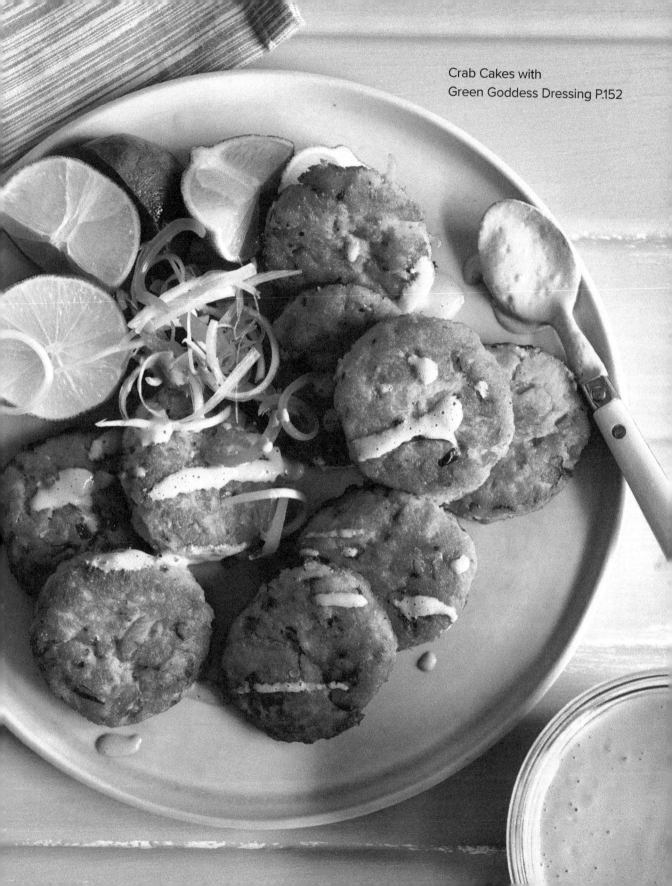

Crab Cakes with
Green Goddess Dressing P.152

Seafood Mains

. . . .

Salmon with Spinach Hemp Pesto

SERVES 4 / PREP TIME: 5 MINUTES / COOK TIME: 20 MINUTES

This salmon and pesto combination creates a perfect keto dish that is high in fat and protein and low enough in carbs to allow any type of side dish. Eating several 4-ounce portions of salmon or other fatty fish, such as mackerel or trout, per week can provide the optimum weekly amount of fish oils—about 300mg.

4 (3-ounce) skinless salmon fillets
½ cup Spinach Hemp Pesto (page 204)

½ lemon, cut into 4 wedges

1. Preheat the oven to 350°F. Line a small baking sheet with aluminum foil.
2. Place the salmon fillets on the baking sheet and spread 2 tablespoons of pesto on each piece of fish. Bake until the fish is opaque, 17 to 20 minutes.
3. Serve with lemon wedges.

Make It Easy: Any pesto is absolutely delicious when used as a salmon topping, so experiment to find your favorite combination. Check the carb and fat content on store-bought pesto, especially sundried tomato pestos, to ensure you are meeting your keto macros.

Per Serving
Macronutrients: Fat: 70 percent; Protein: 30 percent; Carbs: 0 percent
Ketogenic Ratio: 1:1
Calories: 244; Total Fat: 19g; Total Carbohydrates: 1g; Fiber: 1g;
Net Carbs: 0g; Protein: 18g; Sugar Alcohols: 0g

Salmon in Lime Caper Brown Butter Sauce

SERVES 4 / PREP TIME: 10 MINUTES / COOK TIME: 15 MINUTES

Simple can be extraordinary when the ingredients combine so perfectly. Brown butter is an inspired sauce for fish because it is rich, nutty-tasting, and smells heavenly. Take care not to brown it too much or the flavor will turn bitter as the milk solids burn rather than caramelize.

FOR THE SAUCE

½ cup butter, cut into pieces

Juice and zest of 1 lime

1 tablespoon capers

Sea salt

Freshly ground black pepper

FOR THE FISH

4 (4-ounce) salmon fillets

Sea salt

Freshly ground black pepper

2 tablespoons coconut oil

TO MAKE THE SAUCE

1. Place a small saucepan over medium heat and melt the butter. Continue to heat the butter, stirring occasionally, until it is golden brown and very fragrant, about 4 minutes.
2. Remove the brown butter from the heat and stir in the lime zest, lime juice, and capers.
3. Season with salt and pepper and set aside.

Continued on next page

TO MAKE THE FISH

1. Pat the fish dry and season lightly with salt and pepper.
2. Heat the coconut oil in a large skillet over medium-high heat. When the oil is hot, add the salmon and panfry until crispy and golden on both sides, turning once, 6 to 7 minutes per side.
3. Transfer the fish to a serving plate, drizzle with the sauce, and serve.

....

Substitution Tip: Try this recipe with any type of fish, such as tilapia, halibut, or trout.

Per Serving

Macronutrients: Fat: 82 percent; Protein: 18 percent; Carbs: 0 percent

Ketogenic Ratio: 1.9:1

Calories: 485; Total Fat: 44g; Total Carbohydrates: <1g; Fiber: <1g; Net Carbs: 0g; Protein: 23g; Sugar Alcohols: 0g

Roasted Salmon with Black Olive Salsa

SERVES 4 / PREP TIME: 25 MINUTES / COOK TIME: 16 MINUTES

Salsa does not have to be the well-known chopped tomato mixture—this culinary preparation is actually just the Spanish word for sauce. So black olives, sweet sundried tomatoes, and refreshing cucumber and herbs can create a lovely salsa for tender, roasted fish.

FOR THE SALSA

½ cup sliced black olives
½ English cucumber, chopped
¼ cup chopped sundried tomatoes
   packed in oil
1 scallion, white and green parts, chopped
4 tablespoons avocado oil
1 teaspoon chopped fresh basil
1 teaspoon chopped fresh oregano

FOR THE FISH

4 (4-ounce) salmon fillets
2 tablespoons olive oil
Sea salt
Freshly ground black pepper

TO MAKE THE SALSA

1. In a medium bowl, mix together the olives, cucumber, sundried tomatoes, scallion, avocado oil, basil, and oregano.
2. Set aside.

TO MAKE THE FISH

1. Preheat the oven to 350°F. Line a small baking sheet with aluminum foil.
2. Place the fish fillets on the sheet and drizzle them with olive oil.
3. Season the fish lightly with salt and pepper.

Continued on next page

4. Bake the fish until it is opaque, turning once, about 5 minutes per side or until the fish flakes easily with a fork.
5. Serve the fish topped with salsa.

. . . .

Substitution Tip: Salmon is one of the most popular and easiest fish to prepare for home cooks. It is readily available both fresh and frozen. Whenever possible, purchase wild-caught Pacific salmon from Canada or Alaska to avoid mercury contamination.

Per Serving
Macronutrients: Fat: 77 percent; Protein: 21 percent; Carbs: 2 percent
Ketogenic Ratio: 1.4:1
Calories: 457; Total Fat: 39g; Total Carbohydrates: 4g; Fiber: 1g;
Net Carbs: 3g; Protein: 24g; Sugar Alcohols: 0g

Sole with Cucumber Radish Salsa

SERVES 4 / PREP TIME: 15 MINUTES / COOK TIME: 8 MINUTES

This is an attractive dish that screams freshness and summer goodness with the red, white, and green salsa and simple golden pan-fried fish. Sole is one of the most delicate fleshed fish and cooks very quickly, so make sure you supervise that step very closely.

½ English cucumber, chopped

½ avocado, diced

4 radishes, finely chopped

½ scallion, white and green parts, finely chopped

⅓ cup avocado oil, divided

Juice of ½ lemon

1 teaspoon chopped fresh thyme

Sea salt

Freshly ground black pepper

4 (3-ounce) sole fillets

½ cup almond flour

1. In a small bowl, stir together the cucumber, avocado, radish, scallion, 2 tablespoons oil, lemon juice, and thyme.
2. Season with salt and pepper and set aside.
3. Dredge the sole fillets in almond flour.
4. Heat the remaining oil in a large skillet over medium-high heat.
5. Panfry the fish until golden, crispy, and cooked through, turning once, about 8 minutes total.
6. Serve immediately with the cucumber salsa.

Per Serving

Macronutrients: Fat: 72 percent; Protein: 22 percent; Carbs: 6 percent

Ketogenic Ratio: 1.2:1

Calories: 364; Total Fat: 29g; Total Carbohydrates: 7g; Fiber: 3g; Net Carbs: 4g; Protein: 20g; Sugar Alcohols: 0g

Garlic Herb Marinated Tilapia

SERVES 4 / PREP TIME: 10 MINUTES, PLUS TIME TO MARINATE / COOK TIME: 18 MINUTES

Marinated fish with a few citrus wedges is a quick, fuss-free method to cook this delicate protein. Keep in mind that acidic marinades can actually cook the fish, so do not let the fish marinate for longer than about 30 minutes. In half an hour you will add tons of flavor to the fish, and the olive oil will add moisture and prevent any sticking when cooking.

1 cup Garlic Herb Marinade (page 199)
4 (4-ounce) tilapia fillets

Lime wedges

1. Place the marinade in a medium bowl and add the tilapia, turning to coat.
2. Place the bowl, covered, in the refrigerator for 30 minutes.
3. Preheat the oven to 350°F. Line a 9-by-9-inch baking dish with aluminum foil.
4. Arrange the fillets in the baking dish. Pour the marinade over the fish.
5. Bake the fish until it is just cooked through and flaky, 15 to 18 minutes.
6. Serve the tilapia garnished with lime wedges.

Make It Easy: Make the marinade ahead and store in the refrigerator for up to 5 days. When you want to make this meal, simply pour over the fish, marinate, and bake.

Per Serving

Macronutrients: Fat: 76 percent; Protein: 26 percent; Carbs: 1 percent
Ketogenic Ratio: 1.3:1
Calories: 354; Total Fat: 30g; Total Carbohydrates: 2g; Fiber: 1g;
Net Carbs: 1g; Protein: 23g; Sugar Alcohols: 0g

Crispy "Breaded" Fish

SERVES 4 / PREP TIME: 20 MINUTES / COOK TIME: 12 MINUTES

The crunchy golden breading on this flaky haddock is made from spiced almond flour rather than actual bread crumbs, so it suits the keto diet perfectly. Almond flour adds a pleasing sweetness to the already-flavorful fish, and the cardamom has an interesting citrusy, herbal taste.

16 ounces boneless, skinless haddock fillet, cut into 4 pieces
1 cup fine almond flour
½ teaspoon paprika
⅛ teaspoon ground cardamom

⅛ teaspoon sea salt
Pinch freshly ground black pepper
½ cup heavy (whipping) cream
¼ cup coconut oil

1. Rinse the fillets in cold water and pat them completely dry with paper towels.
2. In a medium bowl, stir together the almond flour, paprika, cardamom, salt, and pepper until well blended.
3. Pour the cream into another medium bowl and set it beside the almond flour mixture.
4. Dredge one fish fillet in the flour mixture, shaking off the excess. Then dip the fillet into the cream, shaking off the excess liquid. Finally, dredge the fish in the flour again to coat completely and set aside.
5. Repeat with the remaining fillets.

Continued on next page

6. Place a large skillet over medium-high heat and add the oil.
7. When the oil is hot, place the fillets in the skillet and fry until the fish is golden and crispy, turning once, about 12 minutes total.

· ·

Substitution Tip: If you have an issue with dairy, substitute canned coconut milk or coconut cream for the heavy cream. This will lower the protein macro slightly and increase the fat and carbs, but you will still be within keto ranges.

Per Serving
Macronutrients: Fat: 74 percent; Protein: 24 percent; Carbs: 2 percent
Ketogenic Ratio: 1.2:1
Calories: 475; Total Fat: 39g; Total Carbohydrates: 7g; Fiber: 3g;
Net Carbs: 4g; Protein: 28g; Sugar Alcohols: 0g

Baked Mackerel with Kale and Asparagus

SERVES 4 / PREP TIME: 20 MINUTES / COOK TIME: 15 MINUTES

Packet cooking, or *en papillote,* is an incredibly easy
fish preparation, and success is almost guaranteed because
the fish steams in its own juices and whatever liquid you add.
Mackerel is inexpensive, flavorful, and roasts beautifully with
this method. Be sure to open the packets carefully, because
there will be a lot of hot steam.

2 cups chopped kale

1 cup asparagus, cut into 1-inch pieces

¼ onion, thinly sliced

2 teaspoons chopped fresh basil

4 (3-ounce) mackerel fillets

Sea salt

Freshly ground black pepper

¼ cup olive oil

1 lemon, cut into thin slices

1. Preheat the oven to 400°F.
2. Lay out 4 sheets of aluminum foil, each about 12 inches long.
3. Place ½ cup kale, ¼ cup asparagus, a quarter of the onion slices, and ½ teaspoon of basil in the middle of each piece of foil.
4. Place a fillet on the vegetables and season the fish with salt and pepper.
5. Drizzle the fish with olive oil and arrange lemon slices on top.

Continued on next page

6. Fold the foil up to form loose packets.
7. Set the packets on a baking sheet and bake until the fish is opaque, about 15 minutes.
8. Open the packets carefully and serve.

....

Nutrition Tip: Mackerel is packed with healthy omega-3 fatty acids and no matter which variety you choose, has loads of vitamin B12.

Per Serving

Macronutrients: Fat: 72 percent; Protein: 22 percent; Carbs: 6 percent

Ketogenic Ratio: 1.1:1

Calories: 327; Total Fat: 26g; Total Carbohydrates: 9g; Fiber: 3g;
Net Carbs: 6g; Protein: 18g; Sugar Alcohols: 0g

Rainbow Trout with Cream Leek Sauce

SERVES 4 / PREP TIME: 15 MINUTES / COOK TIME: 17 MINUTES

Trout is a tender, gorgeously pink-fleshed fish with a delicate, almost nutty flavor. You can easily overpower the taste of it, so a light sauce infused with leeks and floral thyme is a perfect accompaniment. Trout is in the same family as keto-friendly salmon, so it should be no surprise that it's high in healthy fats and protein. If you cannot find fresh trout, flash-frozen fillets are a great option.

2 tablespoons olive oil
2 leeks, white and light green parts, thinly sliced and thoroughly washed
1½ cups canned coconut milk

4 (3-ounce) rainbow trout fillets
2 teaspoons chopped fresh thyme
Sea salt
Freshly ground black pepper

1. Heat the olive oil in a large skillet over medium-high heat.
2. Add the leeks and sauté until they are tender, about 7 minutes.
3. Stir in the coconut milk and bring the mixture to a boil.
4. Place the trout in one layer in the liquid and reduce the heat to medium. Simmer until the fish is just cooked through, about 10 minutes.
5. Remove the fillets and place onto 4 plates.

Continued on next page

6. Stir the thyme into the leek cream sauce.
7. Season the sauce with salt and pepper.
8. Spoon the leek sauce over the trout and serve. Please use all of the sauce to ensure the proper fat content.

....

Substitution Tip: Uncured nitrate-free bacon can be added to create an absolutely mouth-watering dish. Panfry 4 pieces of chopped bacon and sauté the leeks in the bacon and its fat instead of olive oil. Prepare the rest of the recipe as directed and enjoy!

Per Serving

Macronutrients: Fat: 75 percent; Protein: 17 percent; Carbs: 8 percent
Ketogenic Ratio: 1.3:1
Calories: 337; Total Fat: 28g; Total Carbohydrates: 9g; Fiber: 1g;
Net Carbs: 8g; Protein: 14g; Sugar Alcohols: 0g

Jambalaya

SERVES 6 / PREP TIME: 20 MINUTES / COOK TIME: 28 MINUTES

Jambalaya gets a keto makeover here with cauliflower standing in for the high-carb grain. Look for okra pods that are firm and plump and have no soft spots or shriveled areas.

⅓ cup olive oil

¼ pound boneless, skinless chicken thighs cut into strips

½ onion, chopped

1 jalapeño pepper, chopped

2 teaspoons minced garlic

1 cup low-sodium chicken stock or Chicken Bone Broth (page 207)

2 cooked Simple Lamb Sausage (page 57) patties or any other cooked sausage, diced

½ pound shrimp, peeled, deveined, and chopped

1 cup okra, cut into ½-inch slices

¼ teaspoon cayenne pepper

3 cups finely chopped cauliflower

Sea salt

Freshly ground black pepper

1. Heat the olive oil in a large skillet over medium-high heat.
2. Sauté the chicken in the oil until just cooked through, about 10 minutes. Remove to a plate using a slotted spoon.
3. Sauté the onion, jalapeño, and garlic until tender, about 3 minutes.
4. Return the chicken breast to the skillet and add the chicken stock, sausage, shrimp, okra, and cayenne. Stir to combine.
5. Bring the mixture to a boil and simmer until the shrimp is cooked and the okra is tender, about 10 minutes. Add the cauliflower and stir until heated through, about 5 minutes.
6. Season with salt and pepper and serve.

Per Serving

Macronutrients: Fat: 70 percent; Protein: 23 percent; Carbs: 7 percent

Ketogenic Ratio: 1.1:1

Calories: 243; Total Fat: 19g; Total Carbohydrates: 6g; Fiber: 2g;

Net Carbs: 4g; Protein: 14g; Sugar Alcohols: 0g

Crab Cakes with Green Goddess Dressing

SERVES 4 / PREP TIME: 15 MINUTES, PLUS TIME TO CHILL / COOK TIME: 17 MINUTES

Crab cakes are famous in the Eastern United States, especially Maryland and Virginia. The best crab cake recipes combine sweet crab meat, a hint of heat, a bit of color, such as red bell pepper, and a fabulous sauce to dip them in. This creation ticks all those culinary boxes. Crab is a great source for protein (about 15 grams in each serving here) and vitamin B12.

5 tablespoons avocado oil, divided

½ red bell pepper, finely chopped

1 scallion, white and green parts, finely chopped

¼ jalapeño pepper, finely chopped

¾ pound real crab meat, shredded

¼ cup almond meal

1 egg

1 teaspoon Dijon mustard

Sea salt

Freshly ground black pepper

½ cup Green Goddess Dressing (page 201)

1. Heat 2 tablespoons of avocado oil in a large skillet over medium-high heat.
2. Sauté the bell pepper, scallion, and jalapeño until softened, about 5 minutes.
3. Transfer the cooked vegetables to a large bowl and add the crab, almond meal, egg, and mustard, mixing until the ingredients are well combined and hold together.

4. Form the crab mixture into 12 patties and place them on a plate, cover with plastic wrap, and chill in the refrigerator to firm for up to 1 hour.
5. Wipe the skillet out and heat the remaining oil over medium-high heat.
6. Panfry the crab cakes until cooked through, about 12 minutes per side, turning once.
7. Season with salt and pepper and top the crab cakes with the dressing and serve.

Substitution Tip: Try adding ½ teaspoon of ground cumin or coriander for a flavor boost.

Per Serving
Macronutrients: Fat: 70 percent; Protein: 22 percent; Carbs: 8 percent
Ketogenic Ratio: 1.3:1
Calories: 358; Total Fat: 28g; Total Carbohydrates: 4g; Fiber: 2g;
Net Carbs: 2g; Protein: 20g; Sugar Alcohols: 0g

Sea Scallops with Curry Sauce

SERVES 4 / PREP TIME: 12 MINUTES / COOK TIME: 18 MINUTES

You can create this elegant dish in about 30 minutes, including the Simple Cauliflower Rice (page 96) to soak up the luscious sauce. Curry pastes come in different colors and flavors—this recipe uses red curry paste made with chili peppers, but you can also try green curry paste (made with cilantro, basil, and kaffir lime leaf) or yellow curry paste (with turmeric).

¾ pound sea scallops, washed, cleaned, and thoroughly dried
Sea salt
Freshly ground black pepper
3 tablespoons olive oil

1 tablespoon peeled, grated fresh ginger
1 to 1½ tablespoons Thai red curry paste
1½ cups canned coconut milk
1 tablespoon chopped fresh cilantro
Zest and juice of 1 lime

1. Season the scallops with salt and pepper.
2. Heat the olive oil in a large skillet over medium-high heat.
3. Pan sear the scallops until browned, about 3 minutes; turn and brown the other side for 3 minutes.
4. Transfer the scallops to a plate, cover loosely with foil, and set aside.
5. Return the skillet to the heat and sauté the ginger until softened, about 2 minutes.
6. Stir in the curry paste, coconut milk, cilantro, lime juice, and lime zest and bring to a simmer for 10 minutes.
7. Reduce the heat to low and return the scallops to the pan, along with any juices on the plate.
8. Turn the scallops with tongs to coat in the sauce and serve.

Per Serving
Macronutrients: Fat: 73 percent; Protein: 19 percent; Carbs: 8 percent
Ketogenic Ratio: 1.2:1
Calories: 334; Total Fat: 27g; Total Carbohydrates: 6g; Fiber: 0g;
Net Carbs: 6g; Protein: 16g; Sugar Alcohols: 0g

Coconut Saffron Mussels

SERVES 4 / PREP TIME: 15 MINUTES / COOK TIME: 12 MINUTES

Plump, flavorful mussels can be a lovely appetizer or part
of the main meal, depending on how you serve them. If you
spoon the mussels and sauce over a portion of cauliflower rice,
you create a tempting entrée.

¼ cup low-sodium vegetable or
   chicken stock
Pinch saffron
3 tablespoons coconut oil
1 scallion, white and green parts,
   thinly sliced
2 teaspoons minced garlic

1 teaspoon peeled, grated fresh ginger
1 cup canned coconut milk
Juice and zest of 1 lime
1½ pounds fresh mussels, scrubbed
   and debearded
2 tablespoons chopped fresh cilantro

1. Put the stock in a small bowl and sprinkle in the saffron. Set aside for 15 minutes.
2. Heat the oil in a large skillet and sauté the scallions, garlic, and ginger until softened, about 3 minutes.
3. Stir in the coconut milk, saffron and liquid, lime juice, and lime zest and bring to a boil.
4. Add the mussels, cover, and steam until the shells are open, about 8 minutes. Discard any unopened shells and take the skillet off the heat.
5. Stir in the cilantro.
6. Serve immediately with the sauce.

Per Serving
Macronutrients: Fat: 80 percent; Protein: 11 percent; Carbs: 9 percent
Ketogenic Ratio: 1.7:1
Calories: 245; Total Fat: 22g; Total Carbohydrates: 7g; Fiber: <1g; Net Carbs: 6g; Protein: 7g;
Sugar Alcohols: 0g

Shrimp Coconut Pad Thai

SERVES 4 / PREP TIME: 20 MINUTES / COOK TIME: 17 MINUTES

Pad Thai didn't originate in Thailand—it is possibly Chinese in origin, brought to Thailand with settlers from southern China. This dish is now served all over the world in many variations. This version has a spicy peanut butter sauce and is just as good cold or warm.

FOR THE SAUCE

1 cup canned coconut milk

¼ cup natural peanut butter

2 tablespoons fish sauce

2 tablespoons apple cider vinegar

2 tablespoons Swerve

1 tablespoon soy sauce

1 tablespoon sriracha hot sauce

FOR THE PAD THAI

4 tablespoons coconut oil

½ pound shrimp, peeled, deveined, and chopped

1 cup bean sprouts

3 zucchini, spiralized

1 scallion, white and green parts, thinly sliced on a bias

TO MAKE THE SAUCE

1. In a medium bowl, whisk together the coconut milk, peanut butter, fish sauce, vinegar, Swerve, soy sauce, and sriracha until smooth.

2. Set aside.

TO MAKE THE PAD THAI

1. Heat the oil in a large skillet over medium-high heat.
2. Sauté the shrimp until just cooked through, about 10 minutes.
3. Add the bean sprouts and sauté 4 minutes.
4. Add the sauce, tossing to coat, and cook until the sauce is heated through, about 3 minutes.
5. Remove from the heat and stir in the zucchini noodles.
6. Serve topped with scallion.

Per Serving

Macronutrients: Fat: 76 percent; Protein: 18 percent; Carbs: 6 percent

Ketogenic Ratio: 1.3:1

Calories: 405; Total Fat: 34g; Total Carbohydrates: 10g; Fiber: 2g; Net Carbs: 8g; Protein: 18g; Sugar Alcohols: 6g

Coconut Ginger Salmon Burgers

SERVES 4 / PREP TIME: 15 MINUTES, PLUS TIME TO CHILL / COOK TIME: 20 MINUTES

Salmon is great for fish burgers because it is meaty, holds up well when barbecued, and tastes marvelous with many interesting flavors. You could add wasabi, black olives, shredded unsweetened coconut, or dill to create different burgers.

12 ounces fresh salmon, chopped

1 egg, beaten

2 tablespoons coconut flour

1 scallion, white and green parts, finely chopped

Juice of 1 lemon

2 teaspoons peeled, grated fresh ginger

½ teaspoon ground coriander

Pinch sea salt

Pinch freshly ground black pepper

4 tablespoons coconut oil

¼ cup Easy Mayonnaise (page 205) or store-bought mayo

1. In a large bowl, combine the salmon, egg, coconut flour, scallion, lemon juice, ginger, coriander, salt, and pepper until well mixed.
2. Form the salmon mixture into 8 equal patties, each ½-inch thick.
3. Chill the salmon patties in the refrigerator until firm, about 1 hour.
4. Heat the oil in a large skillet over medium-high heat.
5. Panfry the salmon burgers, turning once, until cooked through and lightly browned, about 10 minutes per side.
6. Serve 2 burgers per person topped with mayonnaise.

Per Serving

Macronutrients: Fat: 76 percent; Protein: 22 percent; Carbs: 2 percent

Ketogenic Ratio: 1.4:1

Calories: 369; Total Fat: 31g; Total Carbohydrates: 4g; Fiber: 2g; Net Carbs: 2g; Protein: 20g; Sugar Alcohols: 0g

Coconut Milk Baked Haddock

SERVES 4 / PREP TIME: 10 MINUTES / COOK TIME: 27 MINUTES

Haddock is often found in traditional fish and chips because it is a firm-fleshed, sweet, mild fish that can handle thick breading and deep-fat frying. This cold-water fish is high in protein and hearty-healthy fats. Haddock is also a low-mercury fish, so it is appropriate to include regularly in your diet.

2 tablespoons olive oil
1 onion, thinly sliced
1 tablespoon minced garlic
4 (3-ounce) haddock fillets
2 cups canned coconut milk

1 teaspoon ground coriander
½ teaspoon ground cumin
Sea salt
Freshly ground black pepper
2 tablespoons chopped fresh cilantro

1. Preheat the oven to 350°F.
2. Heat the olive oil in a large ovenproof skillet over medium-high heat.
3. Sauté the onion and garlic until lightly caramelized, about 7 minutes.
4. Add the fish to the skillet and brown, turning once, about 8 minutes in total.
5. Add the coconut milk, coriander, and cumin, stirring carefully.
6. Cover and bake until the fish flakes with a fork, about 12 minutes.
7. Season with salt and pepper and serve topped with cilantro.

Substitution Tip: If you do not have an issue with dairy, the traditional cooking method is poaching in milk so that the lactic acid can tenderize the fish. An added benefit is the milk will create its own thick sauce as the protein bakes.

Per Serving
Macronutrients: Fat: 69 percent; Protein: 24 percent; Carbs: 7 percent
Ketogenic Ratio: 1:1
Calories: 381; Total Fat: 29g; Total Carbohydrates: 6g; Fiber: 1g;
Net Carbs: 5g; Protein: 23g; Sugar Alcohols: 0g

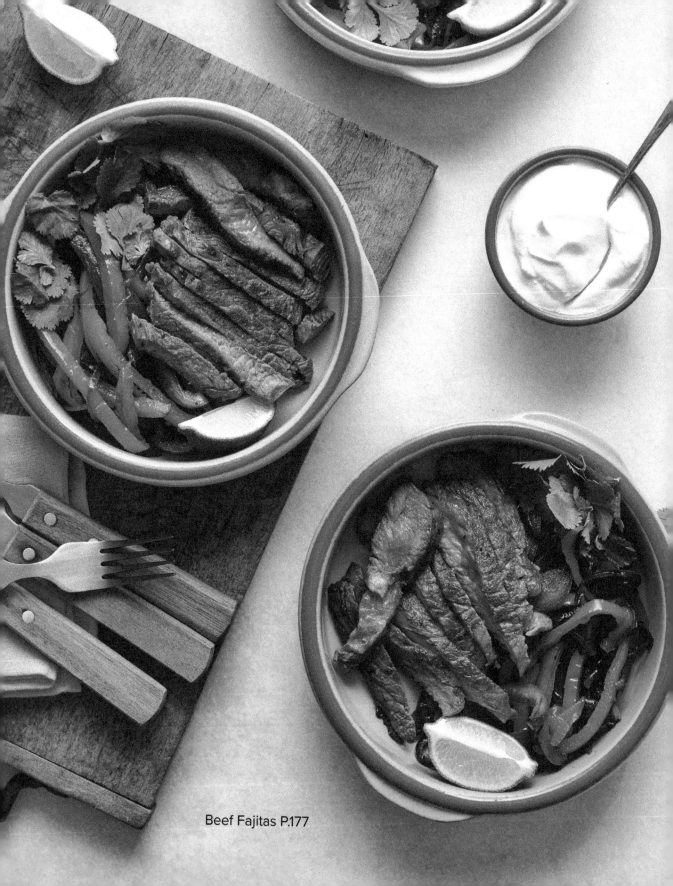

Beef Fajitas P.177

Meaty Mains

. . . .

Chicken Vegetable Hash

SERVES 4 / PREP TIME: 15 MINUTES / COOK TIME: 40 MINUTES

The presentation of this recipe might not be the most attractive and sophisticated you have ever seen, but this dish is tasty and inexpensive. Even if you're not confident in the kitchen, you will have no problem getting a delicious meal on the table. The combination of ingredients adds plenty of antioxidants, vitamins, minerals, healthy fats, and protein to your diet.

¼ cup coconut oil

14 ounces boneless, skinless chicken thighs, diced

1 onion, chopped

1 red bell pepper, diced

2 teaspoons minced garlic

1 cup diced raw or frozen pumpkin

½ cup shredded cabbage

1 teaspoon chopped fresh thyme

Sea salt

Freshly ground black pepper

1 cup pumpkin seeds

½ cup shredded kale

1. Heat the oil in a large skillet over medium-high heat.
2. Sauté the chicken until it is cooked through, about 15 minutes. Transfer the chicken to a plate using a slotted spoon.
3. Add the onion, bell pepper, and garlic and sauté until softened, about 5 minutes.
4. Stir in the pumpkin, cabbage, and thyme and sauté until the vegetables are tender, about 15 minutes.
5. Place the chicken back in the skillet and season with salt and pepper.
6. Add the pumpkin seeds and kale and sauté until the greens are wilted, about 5 minutes.

Per Serving

Macronutrients: Fat: 67 percent; Protein: 23 percent; Carbs: 10 percent

Ketogenic Ratio: 0.9:1

Calories: 443; Total Fat: 33g; Total Carbohydrates: 14g; Fiber: 5g;
Net Carbs: 9g; Protein: 26g; Sugar Alcohols: 0g

Roast Chicken with Cilantro Mayonnaise

SERVES 6 / PREP TIME: 10 MINUTES / COOK TIME: 1 HOUR AND 30 MINUTES

Is there anything more glorious than a perfectly roasted golden chicken, juicy and packed with flavor? Roasted chicken can be a staple in a healthy diet because, once cooked, it can be a satisfying main meal immediately or you can strip the meat off the bones and store it in the refrigerator for salads, soups, and wraps. You can freeze the cooked meat in single-portion bags for up to 3 months.

1 (3-pound) whole roasting chicken
Sea salt, for seasoning
1 onion, cut into 8 wedges
4 tablespoons olive oil

Freshly ground black pepper
½ cup Easy Mayonnaise (page 205), or store-bought mayo
1 tablespoon chopped fresh cilantro

1. Preheat the oven to 350°F.
2. Wash the chicken in cold water, inside and out, and pat it completely dry with paper towels.
3. Place the chicken in a baking dish and lightly salt the cavity.
4. Place the onion in the cavity.
5. Brush the chicken skin all over with olive oil and season the skin with the salt and pepper.
6. Roast the chicken until it is golden brown and cooked through (to an internal temperature of 185°F), about 90 minutes.

Continued on next page

7. Remove the chicken from the oven and let it sit for 15 minutes.
8. In a small bowl, stir together the mayonnaise and cilantro.
9. Carve the chicken and serve with the mayonnaise.

- -

Substitution Tip: The cavity of the chicken is a perfect place to put aromatics designed to flavor the meat, such as lemon and lime halves, and fresh herb sprigs like rosemary, thyme, and sage. You can also place 10 to 12 crushed garlic cloves to create a truly sublime meal.

Per Serving
Macronutrients: Fat: 70 percent; Protein: 30 percent; Carbs: 0 percent
Ketogenic Ratio: 1:1
Calories: 578; Total Fat: 45g; Total Carbohydrates: 4g; Fiber: 1g;
Net Carbs: 3g; Protein: 43g; Sugar Alcohols: 0g

Chicken Cutlets with Garlic Cream Sauce

SERVES 4 / PREP TIME: 20 MINUTES, PLUS TIME TO CHILL / COOK TIME: 25 MINUTES

Cutlets are the base for many traditional recipes, such as chicken and pork schnitzel and chicken Parmesan. This cooking method involves basically pounding the protein to a thinner width, so it cooks faster and evenly when breaded or coated. Coconut and almond are popular keto "breading" and pair well with tender chicken breast. If you want a more delicate flavor, try brushing on avocado oil instead of olive oil.

FOR THE SAUCE
¾ cup canned coconut milk
Juice and zest of 1 lime
1 tablespoon Swerve
2 teaspoons minced garlic
1 teaspoon soy sauce

FOR THE CHICKEN
½ cup almond flour
2 eggs, beaten
¾ cup unsweetened shredded coconut
¼ cup almond meal
4 (3-ounce) boneless, skinless chicken breasts, pounded to about ⅓-inch thick
3 tablespoons olive oil

TO MAKE THE SAUCE
1. Stir together the coconut milk, lime juice, lime zest, Swerve, garlic, and soy sauce in a small saucepan over medium heat.
2. Bring the sauce to a boil, then reduce the heat to low and simmer until thickened, about 5 minutes.
3. Remove the sauce from the heat, pour into a container, and place in the refrigerator until chilled, about 2 hours.

Continued on next page

TO MAKE THE CHICKEN

1. Preheat the oven to 350°F. Line a large baking sheet with parchment paper.
2. Put the almond flour in a small bowl. Put the beaten eggs in another small bowl.
3. In a third bowl, stir together the coconut and almond meal. Line up the bowls with the almond flour, eggs, then the coconut.
4. Pat the chicken dry with paper towels and dredge each piece in the almond flour, then the egg mixture, and finally the coconut mixture to coat.
5. Place the coated chicken on the baking sheet. Brush the cutlets carefully with the olive oil.
6. Bake the chicken until golden brown and cooked through, turning once, about 20 minutes in total.
7. Serve with chilled dipping sauce.

Make It Easy: Freeze the breaded chicken strips on a baking tray then transfer them to a sealed plastic bag and store for up to 2 months in the freezer. Take out the amount you want to serve and bake them from frozen for 35 minutes, turning once.

Per Serving

Macronutrients: Fat: 76 percent; Protein: 20 percent; Carbs: 4 percent
Ketogenic Ratio: 1.3:1
Calories: 508; Total Fat: 43g; Total Carbohydrates: 10g; Fiber: 4g;
Net Carbs: 6g; Protein: 26g; Sugar Alcohols: 3g

Turkey Thyme Burgers

SERVES 4 / PREP TIME: 20 MINUTES / COOK TIME: 25 MINUTES

You do not have to give up burgers because you are following a keto diet—lettuce leaves or grilled Portobello mushrooms work well in place of carb-heavy buns. Pumpkin seeds and coconut are the binders in this tender turkey burger, but you could easily use any low-carb nut flour.

1 pound ground turkey
½ cup ground pumpkin seeds
½ cup shredded unsweetened coconut
1 celery stalk, minced
1 scallion, white and green parts, finely chopped
1 teaspoon minced garlic

1 teaspoon chopped fresh thyme
¼ teaspoon freshly ground black pepper
¼ teaspoon sea salt
¼ cup coconut oil
4 lettuce leaves
2 tablespoons Easy Mayonnaise (page 205), or store-bought mayo

1. Preheat the oven to 350°F. In a large bowl, combine the turkey, pumpkin seeds, coconut, celery, scallion, garlic, thyme, pepper, and salt until uniformly mixed.
2. Form the turkey mixture into 4 patties and flatten them out, so they are about ¾-inch thick.
3. Heat the oil in a large ovenproof skillet over medium-high heat.
4. Brown the turkey burgers, turning once, about 4 minutes per side.
5. Transfer the skillet to the oven and finish cooking until the turkey is cooked through, 15 to 17 minutes.
6. Serve the burgers on lettuce leaves topped with mayo.

Per Serving
Macronutrients: Fat: 74 percent; Protein: 24 percent; Carbs: 2 percent
Ketogenic Ratio: 1.2:1
Calories: 474; Total Fat: 39g; Total Carbohydrates: 7g; Fiber: 3g;
Net Carbs: 4g; Protein: 28g; Sugar Alcohols: 0g

Turkey Pilaf

SERVES 4 / PREP TIME: 15 MINUTES / COOK TIME: 30 MINUTES

Traditionally, pilaf is made with grains and uses a cooking technique that involves finishing the dish in the oven. This particular recipe is not a true pilaf because it uses cauliflower and you will be broiling rather than baking, but the general composition of this recipe holds true. Ground turkey is a very flavorful addition that cooks quickly and adds protein to the dish.

¼ cup coconut oil
¾ pound ground turkey
½ onion, chopped
1 red bell pepper, diced
1 zucchini, diced
2 teaspoons minced garlic
4 cups finely chopped cauliflower

¼ cup chopped fresh parsley
2 tablespoons butter
1 teaspoon chopped fresh thyme
Sea salt
Freshly ground black pepper
1 cup shredded Cheddar cheese

1. Heat the oil in a large ovenproof skillet over medium-high heat.
2. Sauté the ground turkey until cooked through, 12 to 15 minutes. Transfer the meat to a plate using a slotted spoon.
3. Sauté the onion, bell pepper, zucchini, and garlic until softened, about 6 minutes.

4. Stir in the cauliflower, parsley, and cooked turkey and sauté until the cauliflower is tender, about 10 minutes.
5. Preheat the oven to broil.
6. Stir the butter and thyme into the skillet and season everything with salt and pepper.
7. Top the pilaf with the cheese and place the skillet under the broiler until the cheese is melted and bubbly, about 2 minutes.

. . . .

Nutrition Tip: Parsley is an excellent source of vitamin K, and has significant levels of vitamins A and C as well.

Per Serving
Macronutrients: Fat: 70 percent; Protein: 23 percent; Carbs: 7 percent
Ketogenic Ratio: 1.1:1
Calories: 448; Total Fat: 35g; Total Carbohydrates: 11g; Fiber: 4g;
Net Carbs: 7g; Protein: 26g; Sugar Alcohols: 0g

Broiled Lamb Chops with All-Purpose Spice Rub

SERVES 4 / PREP TIME: 10 MINUTES / COOK TIME: 10 MINUTES

Lamb chops come in three different cuts: rib chops, which are from the lamb rack and have a thin bone; shoulder chops, which are the largest and need a bit more cooking time because they are also the toughest; and loin chops, which sit between the other two on the animal and have more meat and are less expensive. You can use any of these cuts for this recipe, with wonderful results.

4 (4-ounce) lamb loin chops, about 1-inch thick

2 tablespoons All-Purpose Spice Rub (page 198)
¼ cup olive oil

1. Rub the lamb chops with the spice rub.
2. Heat the olive oil in a large skillet over medium-high heat.
3. Pan sear the chops until they reach the desired doneness, turning once, about 5 minutes per side for medium-rare.
4. Let the lamb rest 10 minutes before serving.

Nutrition Tip: Lamb is an excellent choice for keto dishes because most cuts are very high in fat, and more than 40 percent is monounsaturated. Lamb is also a great source of niacin, zinc, vitamin B12, and selenium, as well as protein.

Per Serving
Macronutrients: Fat: 85 percent; Protein: 15 percent; Carbs: 0 percent
Ketogenic Ratio: 2.6:1
Calories: 466; Total Fat: 44g; Total Carbohydrates: 1g; Fiber: 1g;
Net Carbs: 0g; Protein: 17g; Sugar Alcohols: 0g

Herb Mustard Lamb Racks

SERVES 4 / PREP TIME: 20 MINUTES / COOK TIME: 20 MINUTES

Lamb racks look spectacular on a plate, especially when arranged bones-up aside a mound of rich Cheesy Mashed Cauliflower (page 98). Frenching lamb racks (removing the meat, fat, and membranes that connect the individual rib bones) can be tricky, but it's worth the effort.

2 frenched lamb racks, 8 bones each
Sea salt
Freshly ground black pepper
¼ cup olive oil, divided
½ cup almond meal

1 tablespoon minced garlic
1 tablespoon chopped fresh rosemary
¼ teaspoon salt
¼ teaspoon freshly ground black pepper
2 tablespoons Dijon mustard

1. Preheat the oven to 450°F.
2. Season the lamb racks with salt and pepper.
3. Heat 2 tablespoons of olive oil in a large ovenproof skillet.
4. Sear the lamb racks on all sides, including the bottom, about 5 minutes total. Remove the skillet from the heat.
5. In a medium bowl, stir together the almond meal, garlic, rosemary, salt, and pepper until well blended. Add the remaining olive oil to the almond mixture, tossing to mix.
6. Spread the mustard on the lamb racks and roll them in the almond mixture.
7. Place the racks back in the skillet bone-side down, and roast until the lamb is the desired doneness, 15 to 18 minutes for medium-rare (125°F to 130°F internal temperature).
8. Let the lamb rest 10 minutes. Cut into serving sizes that are 4 bones each.

Per Serving
Macronutrients: Fat: 77 percent; Protein: 19 percent; Carbs: 4 percent
Ketogenic Ratio: 1.6:1
Calories: 739; Total Fat: 63g; Total Carbohydrates: 7g; Fiber: 2g;
Net Carbs: 5g; Protein: 35g; Sugar Alcohols: 0g

Pork Chops with Mushroom Sauce

SERVES 4 / PREP TIME: 15 MINUTES / COOK TIME: 45 MINUTES

This is a luscious braised dish in which the pork cooks completely immersed in the flavorful mushroom-studded sauce until it is fork-tender. Coconut milk adds a subtle sweetness that is enhanced by fragrant basil. Make sure you eat a quarter of the sauce with each serving to get the full portion of fat!

4 (4-ounce) pork rib chops
Sea salt
Freshly ground black pepper
3 tablespoons olive oil
1 onion, chopped

1 tablespoon minced garlic
4 cups sliced mushrooms
2 cups canned coconut milk
2 teaspoons chopped fresh basil

1. Season the pork chops with salt and pepper.
2. Heat the olive oil in a large skillet over medium-high heat.
3. Pan sear the pork chops on both sides, about 5 minutes per side. Remove the pork chops from the skillet and set aside on a plate.
4. Sauté the onion and garlic until softened, for 3 minutes.

5. Stir in the mushrooms and sauté until they are lightly caramelized, about 10 minutes.

6. Stir in the coconut milk and basil and add the pork chops back to the skillet.

7. Cover the skillet, reduce the heat, and braise until the pork is tender and cooked through, about 20 minutes.

- -

Make It Easy: You can make this scrumptious dish in a slow cooker, after browning the pork rib chops in oil first. Add all the ingredients and cook on low for 8 hours. Be careful when serving if you still have the bones on the pork chops, because they can end up falling off the meat and into the sauce.

Per Serving
Macronutrients: Fat: 71 percent; Protein: 21 percent; Carbs: 8 percent
Ketogenic Ratio: 1.2:1
Calories: 521; Total Fat: 41g; Total Carbohydrates: 8g; Fiber: 1g;
Net Carbs: 7g; Protein: 28g; Sugar Alcohols: 0g

Sriracha Pork Belly

SERVES 4 / PREP TIME: 10 MINUTES, PLUS TIME TO MARINATE / COOK TIME: 3 HOURS

Pork belly comes from exactly the place you would assume—the belly (underside) of the hog. When cured, smoked, and sliced, pork belly becomes bacon. But this cut can be served uncured, so it has none of the triggers associated with migraines and is liberally marbled with fat, which makes it great for a keto diet.

¼ cup sriracha hot sauce

¼ cup no-salt-added tomato paste

2 tablespoons soy sauce

1 tablespoon minced garlic

1 teaspoon Swerve

¾ pound boneless pork belly, with the skin scored

1. In a small bowl, mix together the sriracha, tomato paste, soy sauce, garlic, and Swerve until well combined.
2. Rub half the marinade into the meat part of the pork belly, cover, and marinate for at least 3 hours or overnight.
3. Preheat the oven to 350°F.
4. Place the pork belly skin-side up in a roasting pan, on a wire rack if possible.
5. Roast until the meat is very tender, about 2½ hours.
6. Place the remaining marinade in a small saucepan and cook over medium heat until thick, about 5 minutes.
7. Remove the pork from the oven and lift the crackling (skin) away from the meat.
8. Brush the meat with the glaze and roast for an additional 30 minutes.

Per Serving

Macronutrients: Fat: 85 percent; Protein: 8 percent; Carbs: 7 percent

Ketogenic Ratio: 3:1

Calories: 475; Total Fat: 45g; Total Carbohydrates: 7g; Fiber: 1g; Net Carbs: 6g; Protein: 9g; Sugar Alcohols: 0g

Spicy Pork Wraps

SERVES 4 / PREP TIME: 20 MINUTES

Lettuce wraps allow the complex flavors of the fillings to shine through, and lettuce is readily available and inexpensive. Lettuce is often thought to be a lightweight in the nutrition department, but it is very high in fiber and vitamins A and K. If you cannot get Boston lettuce leaves, try romaine leaves with the rib cut out so the leaf folds, or larger endive leaves.

1 cup shredded fennel

1 cup shredded cucumber, with the liquid squeezed out

1 scallion, white and green parts, chopped

1 tablespoon chopped fresh cilantro

½ recipe Sriracha Pork Belly (page 174), shredded

4 Boston lettuce leaves

½ cup sliced almonds

½ cup crumbled goat cheese

1. In a medium bowl, toss together the fennel, cucumber, scallion, and cilantro until well combined.
2. Divide the pork belly evenly among the lettuce leaves.
3. Top with the fennel mixture, almonds, and goat cheese.
4. Wrap the leaves around the filling by folding over the two opposite sides and then rolling the leaves into cylinders.

Nutrition Tip: Cucumber is an extremely hydrating vegetable—it's about 97 percent water, so it's a stellar choice for a ketogenic diet. It's also very high in vitamin K and contains vitamins A and C, as well as beta-carotene.

Per Serving

Macronutrients: Fat: 80 percent; Protein: 11 percent; Carbs: 9 percent

Ketogenic Ratio: 1.3:1

Calories: 359; Total Fat: 32g; Total Carbohydrates: 9g; Fiber: 4g;

Net Carbs: 5g; Protein: 10g; Sugar Alcohols: 0g

Southwest Meatloaf with Lime Guacamole

SERVES 6 / PREP TIME: 15 MINUTES / COOK TIME: 1 HOUR

Meatloaf is a traditional family meal, created by almost every home cook in some variation and with an assortment of meats and proteins. The ease of preparation and delicious result—good both hot and cold—ensures meatloaf will remain a family favorite. For an extra kick of heat and Southwestern flavor, add half a chopped jalapeño pepper to the mixture.

1 pound ground beef
½ cup almond meal
½ cup chopped onion
½ cup canned coconut milk

1 tablespoon minced garlic
1 tablespoon Southwest seasoning
¼ teaspoon freshly ground black pepper
1 recipe Lime Guacamole (page 206)

1. Preheat the oven to 350°F.
2. In a large bowl, mix together the ground beef, almond meal, onion, coconut milk, garlic, Southwest seasoning, and pepper until very well combined.
3. Pack the meat mixture into a 9-by-4-inch loaf pan.
4. Bake until cooked through and browned, about 1 hour.
5. Let the meatloaf sit for 10 minutes and pour off any accumulated grease.
6. Serve with Lime Guacamole.

Substitution Tip: If you prefer, swap out the ground beef for chicken or pork. You can also use lamb if you like the slightly stronger flavor of this protein.

Per Serving
Macronutrients: Fat: 75 percent; Protein: 17 percent; Carbs: 8 percent
Ketogenic Ratio: 1.5:1
Calories: 396; Total Fat: 33g; Total Carbohydrates: 10g; Fiber: 5g;
Net Carbs: 5g; Protein: 17g; Sugar Alcohols: 0g

Beef Fajitas

SERVES 4 / PREP TIME: 20 MINUTES, PLUS TIME TO MARINATE / COOK TIME: 22 MINUTES

Spicy marinated beef strips and sautéed peppers and onions
wrapped in a lettuce leaf capture the feel of the original. You add a
generous scoop of guacamole and shredded cheese.

¼ cup olive oil, divided
1 tablespoon freshly squeezed lime juice
1 teaspoon ground cumin
1 teaspoon chili powder
1 teaspoon paprika
¼ teaspoon cayenne pepper
Pinch sea salt

Pinch freshly ground black pepper
1 pound boneless rib eye steak
1 red onion, thinly sliced
1 red bell pepper, cut into thin strips
1 green bell pepper, cut into thin strips
2 tablespoons chopped fresh cilantro
½ cup sour cream

1. Put 2 tablespoons of the olive oil, the lime juice, cumin, chili powder, paprika, cayenne, salt, and black pepper in a large resealable plastic bag and shake to combine.
2. Pierce the steak all over with a fork and place the meat in the bag with the marinade. Squeeze out as much air as possible and seal the bag.
3. Marinate the steak for 1 hour in the refrigerator, turning the bag over once.
4. Heat the remaining olive oil in a large skillet over medium-high heat.
5. Pan sear the steak until medium-rare, turning once, 6 to 7 minutes per side.
6. Remove the steak from the heat and let rest for 10 minutes.
7. While the meat rests, sauté the onion and peppers until they are lightly caramelized, about 5 minutes. Remove the vegetables from the heat and stir in the cilantro.
8. Slice the steak thinly on a bias across the grain and serve the meat topped with the vegetable mixture and sour cream.

Per Serving
Macronutrients: Fat: 66 percent; Protein: 22 percent; Carbs: 12 percent
Ketogenic Ratio: 1:1
Calories: 435; Total Fat: 32g; Total Carbohydrates: 11g; Fiber: 2g;
Net Carbs: 9g; Protein: 24g; Sugar Alcohols: 0g

Flank Steak with Kale Chimichurri

SERVES 4 / PREP TIME: 15 MINUTES / COOK TIME: 12 MINUTES

This protein- and flavor-packed meal can be on the table in less than 30 minutes, especially if you serve it with a quick tossed salad or Simple Cauliflower Rice (page 96). Flank steak is a budget-friendly cut of meat that should not be overcooked or it will become tough. Grill or broil it to medium-rare and slice it very thin against the grain for the best results.

½ cup olive oil

½ cup finely chopped kale

2 tablespoons finely chopped fresh parsley

2 tablespoons freshly squeezed lime juice

1 tablespoon minced garlic

1 tablespoon finely chopped fresh chili pepper

½ teaspoon sea salt, plus more for seasoning

½ teaspoon freshly ground black pepper, plus more for seasoning

1 pound flank steak

1. To make the chimichurri, in a medium bowl, stir together the olive oil, kale, parsley, lime juice, garlic, chili pepper, salt, and pepper until well combined. Set aside.
2. Preheat the barbecue to medium-high heat.
3. Lightly season both sides of the steak with salt and pepper.
4. Grill the steak 5 to 6 minutes per side for medium-rare.
5. If you do not have a barbecue, preheat the oven to broil and broil the steak until it is the desired doneness, 5 to 6 minutes per side for medium-rare.
6. Let the steak rest for 10 minutes before slicing it thinly across the grain.
7. Serve with the chimichurri.

Per Serving

Macronutrients: Fat: 74 percent; Protein: 23 percent; Carbs: 3 percent

Ketogenic Ratio: 1.3:1

Calories: 426; Total Fat: 35g; Total Carbohydrates: 2g; Fiber: 0g;

Net Carbs: 2g; Protein: 25g; Sugar Alcohols: 0g

Butter-Basted Rib Eye Steaks

SERVES 4 / PREP TIME: 10 MINUTES, PLUS TIME TO MARINATE / COOK TIME: 15 MINUTES

If you are a fan of cooking shows, you will have seen some professional chef butter-basting a steak in a massive cast iron skillet. This
is a classic method for preparing steak and can be duplicated easily
at home without the cast iron. Butter-basting adds flavor, but it also
creates a lovely brown crust on the meat, because the milk solids in
the butter caramelize and the butter seeps into the meat. Delicious!

2 (¾-pound) bone-in rib eye steaks
Sea salt
Freshly ground black pepper
1 tablespoon olive oil

¼ cup butter
1 teaspoon chopped fresh thyme
4 garlic cloves, crushed

1. Season the rib eye steaks with salt and pepper. Let the steaks sit at room temperature for
   30 minutes.
2. Heat the olive oil in a large skillet, cast iron if possible, over high heat.
3. Pan sear the steaks until brown and crusty on the bottom, 5 to 6 minutes. Flip the steaks
   and add the butter, thyme, and garlic to the skillet.
4. Cook the steaks, basting with the melted butter, garlic, and herbs, until the steaks are
   medium-rare, 6 to 8 minutes more.
5. Let the steaks rest 10 minutes on a cutting board and slice them across the grain.

Substitution Tip: This is a classic steak preparation, creating flavorful, rich, crusted beef
infused with garlic and herbs. Try rosemary, marjoram, tarragon, or oregano along with or
instead of the thyme sprigs for a delicious variation.

Per Serving
Macronutrients: Fat: 84 percent; Protein: 33 percent; Carbs: 1 percent
Ketogenic Ratio: 1.1:1
Calories: 474; Total Fat: 44g; Total Carbohydrates: 1g; Fiber: 0g;
Net Carbs: 1g; Protein: 39g; Sugar Alcohols: 0g

Moussaka

SERVES 6 / PREP TIME: 25 MINUTES / COOK TIME: 1 HOUR AND 25 MINUTES

Moussaka is a traditional Greek casserole consisting of layers—eggplant, beef, tomato sauce, creamy sauce, and cheese in this recipe. Although the coconut milk–based sauce is not a real béchamel, you will still get a very close version of the original famous dish. This dish freezes well either unbaked or baked, so double up the recipe for a future quick meal.

1 eggplant, cut into 1-inch rounds

3 tablespoons olive oil, divided

1 pound ground beef

1 onion, chopped

2 teaspoons minced garlic

1 cup no-sugar-added tomato sauce

¼ cup low-sodium beef stock or Beef Bone Broth (page 208)

¼ cup almond meal

2 tablespoons chopped fresh parsley

2 eggs

½ teaspoon sea salt

½ teaspoon freshly ground black pepper

3 tablespoons melted butter

1 cup canned coconut milk

1 cup shredded mozzarella cheese, divided

¼ teaspoon ground nutmeg

1. Preheat the oven to 375°F.
2. Place the eggplant in a single layer on a large baking sheet and brush with 2 tablespoons of the olive oil.
3. Roast the eggplant in the oven until softened, about 10 minutes. Remove from the oven and let cool.
4. Heat the remaining olive oil in a large skillet over medium-high heat. Brown the beef until completely cooked through, 12 to 15 minutes.

5. Add the onion and garlic and sauté for 3 minutes.
6. Stir in the tomato sauce and beef stock and bring the sauce to a boil. Reduce the heat to low and simmer for 10 minutes.
7. Let the sauce cool for 15 minutes, then stir in the almond meal, parsley, eggs, salt, and pepper. This is the meat sauce.
8. While the meat sauce is cooling, in a medium saucepan over medium heat, whisk together the butter, coconut milk, ½ cup of the cheese, and nutmeg. Stir until the cheese is melted and the sauce is thick, about 4 minutes. This is the cheese sauce.
9. Place half the eggplant rounds in a 9-by-13-inch baking dish and top with the meat sauce.
10. Layer the remaining eggplant rounds on top of the meat sauce and pour the cheese sauce over them.
11. Sprinkle the remaining mozzarella cheese on top and bake until bubbly and heated through, about 45 minutes.

Make It Easy: You can make this casserole ahead of time and store it in the refrigerator for up to 2 days before baking it. You can also freeze the moussaka for up to 1 month and bake right from frozen. Just add about 30 minutes to the cook time.

Per Serving
Macronutrients: Fat: 74 percent; Protein: 19 percent; Carbs: 7 percent
Ketogenic Ratio: 1.2:1
Calories: 513; Total Fat: 42g; Total Carbohydrates: 14g; Fiber: 4g;
Net Carbs: 10g; Protein: 24g; Sugar Alcohols: 0g

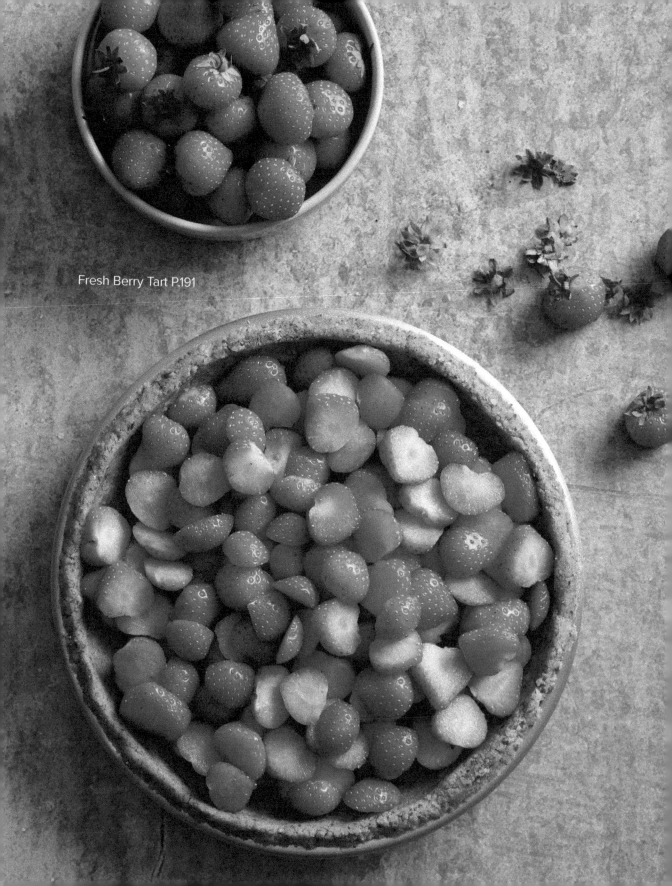

Fresh Berry Tart P.191

Desserts

. . . .

Grilled Cantaloupe

SERVES 4 / PREP TIME: 15 MINUTES / COOK TIME: 10 MINUTES

Fruit is the perfect ingredient to grill when you want a simple dessert with some impact. Most high-sugar fruits such as peaches and pineapple are the best to grill because they caramelize so beautifully, but these choices are very limited on the keto diet. Luckily, cantaloupe is equally delicious grilled or broiled. Make sure your cantaloupe is ripe but not too soft or you will not be able to turn it as it heats up.

1 small cantaloupe, cut into 1-inch-thick slices, seeded, with the rind intact
2 tablespoons melted coconut oil
½ teaspoon ground cinnamon

Pinch ground cloves
Pinch sea salt
½ cup heavy (whipping) cream

1. Preheat the barbecue to medium and clean the grill very well. Or preheat a grill pan on the stovetop.
2. Brush the cut edges of the melon with coconut oil.
3. Sprinkle the slices with cinnamon, cloves, and salt.

4. Grill the melon slices until they are tender and very lightly charred, turning once, about 10 minutes total.
5. Transfer the melon to a plate and set aside.
6. Whip the cream until fluffy and thick, about 5 minutes.
7. Serve the grilled cantaloupe with whipped cream.

Substitution Tip: Lactose is a common allergy, so instead of heavy cream, whip up coconut cream. You can either buy an entire can of coconut cream and chill it, or scoop the coconut cream off the top of a can of chilled full-fat coconut milk. Then beat it with an electric hand beater until it's the perfect texture.

Per Serving
Macronutrients: Fat: 80 percent; Protein: 4 percent; Carbs: 16 percent
Ketogenic Ratio: 1.6:1
Calories: 201; Total Fat: 18g; Total Carbohydrates: 10g; Fiber: 1g;
Net Carbs: 9g; Protein: 2g; Sugar Alcohols: 0g

Blueberry Mint Ice Pops

Ice pops can be a simple children's treat or a more sophisticated adult dessert on a balmy summer evening. This recipe falls somewhere in between, with its minty, lightly sweetened berry flavor and added freshness from the cucumber. For an extremely smooth texture, you can pour the blended mixture through a fine sieve to remove bits of mint and cucumber peel. Or you can leave the dark green bits in to add an interesting appearance to the pops.

2 cups blueberries
1 English cucumber, cut into chunks
1 cup heavy (whipping) cream

2 teaspoons Swerve
¼ cup fresh mint
Pinch ground nutmeg

1. Place the blueberries, cucumber, cream, Swerve, mint, and nutmeg in a blender and pulse until the mixture is very smooth.
2. Pour the mixture into ice pop molds and freeze until firm.
3. Serve.

Substitution Tip: Basil can replace the mint in these pretty pops if you like the subtle licorice flavor.

Per Serving
Macronutrients: Fat: 72 percent; Protein: 5 percent; Carbs: 23 percent
Ketogenic Ratio: 1.4:1
Calories: 87; Total Fat: 7g; Total Carbohydrates: 5g; Fiber: 1g;
Net Carbs: 4g; Protein: 1g; Sugar Alcohols: 1g

Mixed Berry Sherbet

SERVES 6 / PREP TIME: 15 MINUTES, PLUS 6 HOURS TO FREEZE

Sherbet, sorbet, granita, gelato, and ice cream—it is hard sometimes to keep straight which dish is which when considering a scrumptious frozen treat. Sherbet, unlike sorbet, contains dairy or some sort of dairy substitute to create creaminess, similar to ice cream. This recipe is called sherbet because of the addition of coconut milk, but real sherbet can contain only 2 percent fat, so it misses the mark. No matter what it's called, dig in and enjoy!

3 cups berries (aim for a mixture of strawberries, raspberries, blueberries, and blackberries)

2 cups canned coconut milk

6 ounces firm tofu

1 tablespoon Swerve

1 tablespoon chopped fresh thyme

1. Place the berries, coconut milk, tofu, Swerve, and thyme in a food processor or blender and process until smooth.
2. Press the mixture through a fine sieve to remove the seeds.
3. Pour the mixture into a 9-by-13-inch metal baking dish.
4. Place the baking dish in the freezer for 3 hours.
5. Stir the partially frozen mixture, scraping the sides, then return the container to the freezer.
6. Scrape the sides and bottom with a fork or spoon every hour until it starts to freeze solid, about 6 hours.

Continued on next page

7. When you are ready to serve, use a fork to scrape until the mixture is the texture of snow.
8. Store the sherbet in a sealed container in the freezer for up to 1 month, scraping whenever you want to serve it.

Nutrition Tip: Berries are incredibly high in phytonutrients and anti-inflammatories, as well vitamins C and K and manganese. They provide trace amounts of numerous other vitamins and minerals that make them a great way to "spend" a few of your carbs on a keto diet!

Per Serving
Macronutrients: Fat: 72 percent; Protein: 8 percent; Carbs: 20 percent
Ketogenic Ratio: 1.4:1
Calories: 289; Total Fat: 23g; Total Carbohydrates: 15g; Fiber: 4g;
Net Carbs: 11g; Protein: 6g; Sugar Alcohols: 2g

Strawberry Avocado Ice Cream

SERVES 6 / PREP TIME: 10 MINUTES, PLUS 6 HOURS TO FREEZE

Avocado and strawberries combine as a lovely, rich base for this cool, decadent dessert. The sweetness of the strawberries is highlighted by vanilla and a hint of warm nutmeg. Try serving this on a slice of Fresh Berry Tart (page 191) for a lovely treat.

3 cups halved strawberries
1 ripe avocado, chopped
½ cup heavy (whipping) cream
½ cup plain Greek yogurt

2 teaspoons Swerve
½ teaspoon vanilla extract
¼ teaspoon ground nutmeg

1. Place the strawberries, avocado, cream, yogurt, Swerve, vanilla, and nutmeg in a food processor or blender and purée until smooth.
2. If you want very smooth ice cream, pass the mixture through a fine sieve to remove the seeds.
3. Pour the mixture into a 9-by-13-inch metal baking dish and freeze it solid, about 6 hours.
4. Just before serving, transfer the frozen mixture to a blender or food processor and pulse until it resembles soft ice cream. Only transfer the amount you wish to serve because you can only do this process once.
5. Serve immediately after blending.
6. Store the remaining frozen mixture in the freezer for up to one month in a sealed freezer bag.

Per Serving
Macronutrients: Fat: 70 percent; Protein: 5 percent; Carbs: 25 percent
Ketogenic Ratio: 1.3:1
Calories: 166; Total fat: 13g; Total Carb: 12g; Fiber: 4g;
Net Carb: 8g; Protein: 2g; Sugar Alcohols: 2g

Double Coconut Panna Cotta

SERVES 4 / PREP TIME: 20 MINUTES, PLUS 4 HOURS TO SET / COOK TIME: 20 MINUTES

Panna cotta is one of the simplest desserts to make and is incredibly versatile, so you can use any type of milk in the preparation. Coconut milk is used here to provide fat and flavor to the dish as well as fiber.

2¼ teaspoons unflavored powdered gelatin
¼ cup cold water
3 cups canned coconut milk

1 tablespoon Swerve
2 teaspoons vanilla extract
½ cup shredded unsweetened coconut

1. In a small bowl, sprinkle the gelatin into the water and let stand for 10 to 15 minutes to soften. Then stir until dissolved.
2. In a large saucepan, heat the coconut milk, Swerve, and vanilla over medium heat until scalded but not boiling.
3. Remove the coconut milk mixture from the heat and whisk in the gelatin.
4. Pour the mixture into 4 serving dishes and chill until set, 3 to 4 hours.
5. Preheat the oven to 325°F.
6. Spread the shredded coconut on a baking sheet in a thin layer and bake until toasted and golden, stirring a few times, 5 to 10 minutes. Cool the coconut completely.
7. Serve the panna cotta topped with toasted coconut.

Substitution Tip: Create a luscious chocolate dessert by adding 2 tablespoons of cacao powder to the coconut milk mixture and increasing the sweetener by 2 teaspoons. Cacao powder is rich in migraine-fighting magnesium and is an effective antioxidant. Look for high-fat Dutch-style cacao for the best taste and texture.

Per Serving
Macronutrients: Fat: 81 percent; Protein: 9 percent; Carbs: 10 percent
Ketogenic Ratio: 2.3:1
Calories: 340; Total Fat: 32g; Total Carbohydrates: 9g; Fiber: 2g;
Net Carbs: 7g; Protein: 7g; Sugar Alcohols: 3g

Fresh Berry Tart

SERVES 6 / PREP TIME: 20 MINUTES, PLUS TIME TO CHILL

Who knew pie could be so quick and easy to prepare? This dessert was designed as a raw vegan alternative to regular pies, and the tempting crust can be filled with an assortment of berries if strawberries are not in season. The quality and taste of the berries are crucial for the best dessert. Strawberries are very perishable, and if you leave them in the refrigerator for more than two days, they will start losing precious vitamin C.

½ cup chopped pecans
½ cup almond flour
¼ cup coconut oil

¼ teaspoon ground cinnamon
4 cups sliced strawberries

1. Place the pecans, almond flour, coconut oil, and cinnamon in a blender and pulse until the mixture holds together and is well mixed.
2. Press the nut mixture into an 8-inch pie plate and chill until firm.
3. Fill the crust with fresh berries and serve immediately.

Nutrition Tip: Strawberries are incredibly healthy and delicious, especially in season. They are rich in ellagic acid, a micronutrient with antioxidant properties. One serving of this lovely dessert will nearly meet your vitamin C needs for the day!

Per Serving
Macronutrients: Fat: 81 percent; Protein: 7 percent; Carbs: 13 percent
Ketogenic Ratio: 2.1:1
Calories: 234; Total Fat: 21g; Total Carbohydrates: 11g; Fiber: 5g;
Net Carbs: 6g; Protein: 4g; Sugar Alcohols: 0g

Creamy Lemon Cheesecake

SERVES 12 / PREP TIME: 20 MINUTES, PLUS TIME TO COOL / COOK TIME: 1 HOUR AND 10 MINUTES

Cheesecake is quite possibly the most decadent, luscious dessert ever created, with its dense creaminess and plethora of flavors. The trick to making a perfect cheesecake is beating the ingredients. You must beat the cream cheese until it is absolutely smooth or you will never get the lumps out after adding the other ingredients. Make sure you scrape down the sides of the bowl well after adding every ingredient, even individual eggs, and your cheesecake will be incredible. You cannot rush the preparation of this beautiful dessert.

2 cups almond flour

3 tablespoons coconut oil

32 ounces cream cheese, at room temperature

⅔ cup Swerve

4 eggs, at room temperature

½ cup sour cream

Juice and zest of 1 lemon

1 teaspoon vanilla extract

1. Preheat the oven to 350°F.
2. Place a 9-inch springform pan on a large piece of aluminum foil and wrap the foil up the sides of the pan.
3. In a medium bowl, stir together the almond flour and coconut oil until the mixture resembles coarse crumbs. Press the almond mixture into the bottom of the pan to form an even layer.
4. Bake the crust until firm, about 10 minutes. Cool the crust completely.

5. Increase the oven temperature to 425°F.
6. In a large bowl, beat together the cream cheese and Swerve until very smooth, scraping down the sides of the bowl often.
7. Beat in the eggs one at a time, scraping down the sides of the bowl after each addition.
8. Beat in the sour cream, lemon juice, lemon zest, and vanilla.
9. Pour the cheesecake batter into the crust and bake for 10 minutes, then lower the temperature to 225°F.
10. Bake until the sides are set, about 1 hour. Turn off the oven and cool the cheesecake in the oven to room temperature.
11. Refrigerate the cheesecake overnight, covered in plastic wrap.

Substitution Tip: This is a marvelous base cheesecake, which can be topped with fresh berries, unsweetened chocolate, and nuts. You can stir these flavorful ingredients right into the batter, as well, and bake using the same time and method.

Per Serving
Macronutrients: Fat: 87 percent; Protein: 11 percent; Carbs: 3 percent
Ketogenic Ratio: 2.4:1
Calories: 445; Total Fat: 43g; Total Carbohydrates: 8g; Fiber: 2g;
Net Carbs: 6g; Protein: 12g; Sugar Alcohols: 12g

Rich Pumpkin Mousse

SERVES 6 / PREP TIME: 15 MINUTES, PLUS 1 HOUR TO CHILL

Pumpkin will always seem like an autumn fruit to most people in North America, so warm spices like cinnamon and nutmeg are a natural accompaniment. Cinnamon is rich in vitamin K, calcium, magnesium, iron, and manganese.

2 tablespoons unflavored powdered gelatin
1 cup heavy (whipping) cream, divided
2 cups puréed pumpkin
1 avocado, cut into quarters

1 tablespoon Swerve
½ teaspoon ground cinnamon
¼ teaspoon ground nutmeg
Pinch ground cloves

1. In a small bowl, sprinkle the gelatin on ¼ cup cream and let stand for 10 minutes to dissolve.
2. Place the remaining cream, gelatin mixture, pumpkin, avocado, Swerve, cinnamon, nutmeg, and cloves in a food processor and purée until silky smooth.
3. Spoon the mousse into 6 serving bowls and place them in the refrigerator for 1 hour to set.

Substitution Tip: If you want a vegan mousse, swap out the heavy cream for canned coconut milk or coconut cream and substitute an equal amount of powdered agar-agar for the gelatin. Bring all the coconut milk and agar-agar to a boil in a small saucepan, then simmer for 2 minutes. Remove from the heat and add to the other ingredients in the blender. Then proceed with the recipe.

Per Serving
Macronutrients: Fat: 81 percent; Protein: 9 percent; Carbs: 10 percent
Ketogenic Ratio: 2:1
Calories: 221; Total Fat: 20g; Total Carbohydrates: 10g; Fiber: 5g;
Net Carbs: 5g; Protein: 5g; Sugar Alcohols: 4g

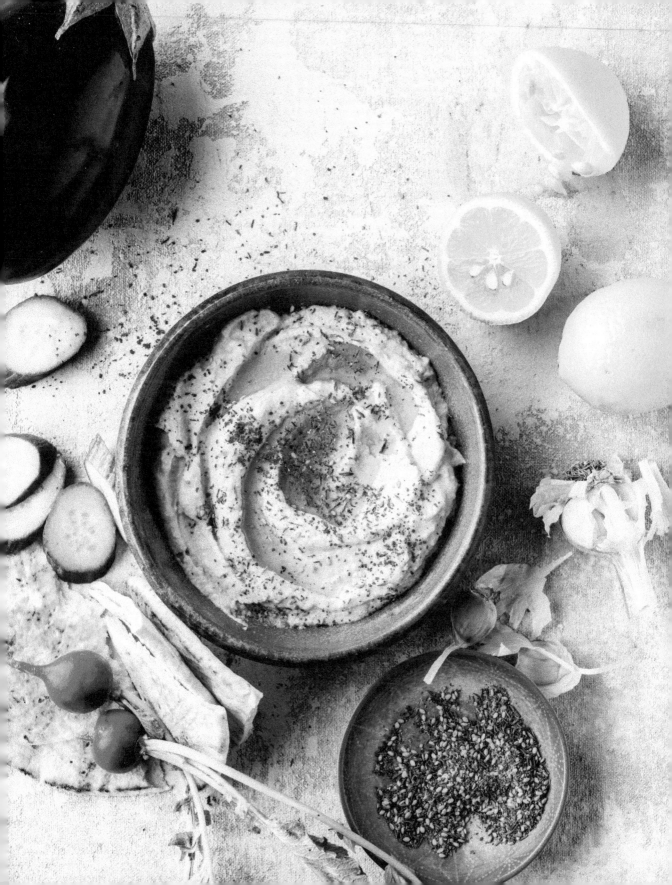

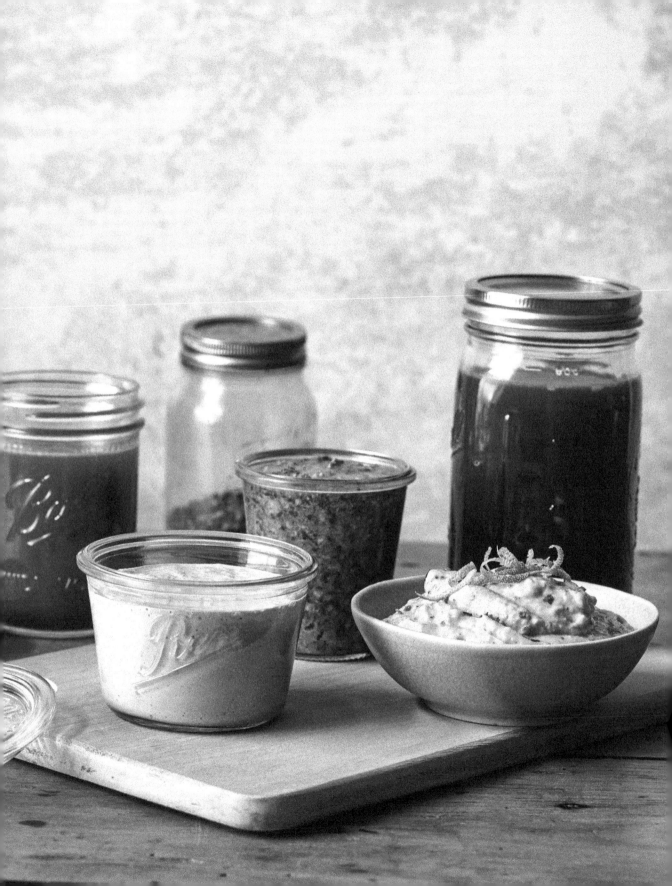

CHAPTER 12

Staples

. . . .

All-Purpose Spice Rub

MAKES ¾ CUP / PREP TIME: 5 MINUTES

There is a dizzying array of spice blends in your local grocery store, so you might be wondering why you should make your own. Creating the perfect mixture of spices and dried herbs can elevate your cooking to another level, and everyone's palate is different. So experimenting with these ingredients can be fun and the results satisfying. Start with the base recipe here and adjust it as you see fit.

4 tablespoons celery salt
4 tablespoons dried thyme
2 tablespoons dried oregano

1 tablespoon freshly ground black pepper
1 tablespoon smoked paprika
2 teaspoons ground coriander

1. Stir together the celery salt, thyme, oregano, pepper, paprika, and coriander in a small bowl until well combined.
2. Transfer the spice mixture to a sealed container and store it in a cool, dark place for up to 2 months.

Substitution Tip: The type of spices and amount are flexible in this mixture, so experiment to create your favorite combinations. Cumin, marjoram, basil, red pepper flakes, Himalayan sea salt, and rosemary would all be nice additions.

Per Serving (1 tablespoon)
Macronutrients: Fat: 50 percent; Protein: 22 percent; Carbs: 28 percent
Ketogenic Ratio: 0.5:1
Calories: 18; Total Fat: 1g; Total Carbohydrates: 3g; Fiber: 2g;
Net Carbs: 1g; Protein: 1g; Sugar Alcohols: 0g

Garlic Herb Marinade

MAKES 1 CUP / PREP TIME: 15 MINUTES

There are usually two types of home cooks: those who use marinades and those who do not. If you are new to marinades, the depth of flavor this herb and flavor-packed recipe can produce in proteins will please you. Depending on the amount of meat, poultry, or fish you are making, you can set use ¼ cup of the marinade to baste the proteins when barbecuing or roasting. This will intensify the taste even more.

½ cup olive oil
Juice and zest of ½ lemon
Juice and zest of ½ lime
1½ teaspoons minced garlic

2 teaspoons chopped fresh basil
2 teaspoons chopped fresh thyme
1 teaspoon chopped fresh oregano
¼ teaspoon sea salt

1. Whisk together the olive oil, lemon and lime juices and zests, garlic, basil, thyme, oregano, and salt in a medium bowl until well combined.
2. Store the marinade in the refrigerator in a sealed container until you want to use it, up to 1 week.

Substitution Tip: Try using roasted garlic instead of fresh for a rich flavor. Toss 12 garlic cloves with 1 tablespoon of olive oil in a small ovenproof skillet and roast, covered, in a 350°F oven until very tender and lightly caramelized, about 25 minutes.

Per Serving (2 tablespoons)
Macronutrients: Fat: 97 percent; Protein: 0 percent; Carbs: 3 percent
Ketogenic Ratio: 14:1
Calories: 122; Total Fat: 14g; Total Carbohydrates: 1g; Fiber: 0g;
Net Carbs: 1g; Protein: 0g; Sugar Alcohols: 0g

Lemon Poppy Seed Dressing

MAKES 1¾ CUPS / PREP TIME: 5 MINUTES

Sweet, tart, and with an interesting texture from the generous amount of poppy seeds, this dressing works for everything from mixed green salads to coleslaw. You can adjust the sweetener depending on your own taste, but make sure you use the Swerve that is 1:1 with sugar. For an extra lemon kick, you can add 1 teaspoon of lemon zest as well.

1 cup olive oil
½ cup freshly squeezed lemon juice
2 tablespoons apple cider vinegar

2 tablespoons Swerve
1 tablespoon poppy seeds
Sea salt

1. Place the olive oil, lemon juice, vinegar, Swerve, and poppy seeds in a medium bowl and whisk to combine well.
2. Season with salt.
3. Pour into a container and store the dressing in the refrigerator for up to 2 weeks.
4. Take the dressing out of the refrigerator about 10 minutes before you want to use it, and shake well before pouring it on your salad.

Nutrition Tip: Olive oil is an essential component of any ketogenic diet. This monounsaturated fat provides omega-3 fatty acids and the antioxidant CoQ10.

Per Serving (2 tablespoons)
Macronutrients: Fat: 100 percent; Protein: 0 percent; Carbs: 0 percent
Ketogenic Ratio: 15:1
Calories: 142; Total Fat: 16g; Total Carbohydrates: 1g; Fiber: <1g;
Net Carbs: <1g; Protein: <1g; Sugar Alcohols: 2g

Green Goddess Dressing

This dressing sounds very "spring in a country garden," and it's appropriately named because the mixture is very green and herbal, with a hint of citrus and sweetness. If you have a dietary issue with citrus, increase the apple cider vinegar to ¼ cup and leave out the lemon juice.

1 avocado, peeled
½ cup fresh basil
1 scallion, white and green parts, chopped
¼ cup extra-virgin olive oil
¼ cup chopped fresh parsley
Juice of 1 large lemon

2 tablespoons apple cider vinegar
2 teaspoons Swerve
1 teaspoon minced garlic
¼ teaspoon sea salt
Water, to thin the dressing

1. In a food processor, pulse the avocado, basil, scallion, olive oil, parsley, lemon juice, vinegar, Swerve, garlic, and salt until blended.
2. If the dressing is too thick, add some water a little bit at a time.
3. Refrigerate in a sealed container for up to 2 weeks.

Nutrition Tip: Basil is one of the most popular herbs in the world because of its delightful flavor.

Per Serving (2 tablespoons)
Macronutrients: Fat: 90 percent; Protein: <1 percent; Carbs: 9 percent
Ketogenic Ratio: 5:1
Calories: 50; Total Fat: 5g; Total Carbohydrates: 1g; Fiber: 1g;
Net Carbs: 0g; Protein: <1g; Sugar Alcohols: 0g

Classic Hollandaise

MAKES 2 CUPS / PREP TIME: 20 MINUTES / COOK TIME: 20 MINUTES

Don't be afraid to attempt this classic French sauce—it's not as hard as it looks, and the results are sublime. The trick to a good hollandaise is to cook your egg yolks but not let them solidify. This classic technique creates a spectacular sauce, but you can do it in a blender with good results if you are not concerned about raw eggs. Follow this recipe to step 2, then place the yolks, water, and lemon juice in a blender and blend on high for 5 seconds. Unsnap the cap on the blender (not the lid) and slowly pour in the melted butter while the blender runs on high speed. Season with salt and serve immediately.

1½ cups unsalted butter
4 egg yolks
1 teaspoon cold water

1 tablespoon freshly squeezed lemon juice
Pinch sea salt

1. Melt the butter in a medium saucepan over low heat.
2. Remove the saucepan from the heat and let sit for 10 minutes, then skim off any foam from the top.
3. Pour the clear yellow (clarified) butter from the saucepan, leaving the milky solids in the pan. Set the clarified bitter aside for 30 minutes to cool.
4. Place a medium saucepan with about 3 inches of water over medium heat until the water simmers gently.

5. Whisk the yolks in a large stainless steel bowl with 1 teaspoon of cold water until light and foamy, about 4 minutes.
6. Reduce the heat under the simmering water to low and place the bowl with the eggs onto the saucepan, making sure the bottom of the bowl does not touch the simmering water.
7. Whisk the yolks until they thicken, about 2 minutes, then remove the bowl from the simmering saucepan.
8. Add the clarified butter to the yolk mixture in a thin stream, whisking continuously, until the sauce is thick and smooth and all the butter is used up.
9. Whisk in the lemon juice and season with salt.
10. Use the sauce immediately.

Substitution Tip: Add ¼ cup of chopped fresh tarragon to the finished hollandaise to create a béarnaise sauce to use with seafood, eggs, and vegetables. Tarragon has a gorgeous, licorice-like flavor that's popular in French cooking.

Per Serving (2 tablespoons)
Macronutrients: Fat: 97 percent; Protein: 2 percent; Carbs: <1 percent
Ketogenic Ratio: 18:1
Calories: 167; Total Fat: 18g; Total Carbohydrates: <1g; Fiber: 0g;
Net Carbs: 0g; Protein: 1g; Sugar Alcohols: 0g

Spinach Hemp Pesto

MAKES 2 CUPS / PREP TIME: 15 MINUTES

Pesto is one of those condiments you always need on hand because of its incredible range of uses. This version has dark leafy greens, herbs, garlic, lemon, and hemp hearts to boost the nutrition profile. You could just as easily make it with only herbs, pine nuts or pecans, and a generous amount of Parmesan cheese to create a more traditional pesto. Experiment to find your favorite ingredients.

1 cup spinach
1 cup fresh basil
½ cup fresh oregano
¼ cup hemp hearts
2 tablespoons freshly squeezed lemon juice

2 garlic cloves
½ cup extra-virgin olive oil
Sea salt
Freshly ground black pepper

1. Place the spinach, basil, oregano, hemp hearts, lemon juice, and garlic in a blender and pulse until the mixture is very finely chopped.
2. Drizzle in the olive oil in a thin stream while the blender is running, until all the oil is added.
3. Scrape down the sides of the blender and pulse until the pesto is the desired texture.
4. Season with salt and pepper.
5. Store the pesto in a sealed container in the refrigerator for up to 2 weeks.

Nutrition Tip: Hemp hearts have a rich nutritional profile, including a nice amount of protein—about 10 grams per 3 tablespoons.

Per Serving (2 tablespoons)
Macronutrients: Fat: 92 percent; Protein: 5 percent; Carbs: 3 percent
Ketogenic Ratio: 8:1
Calories: 78; Total Fat: 8g; Total Carbohydrates: 1g; Fiber: 1g;
Net Carbs: 0g; Protein: 1g; Sugar Alcohols: 0g

Easy Mayonnaise

Mayonnaise is one of the simpler sauces to create at home, as it's an emulsion that just requires some whisking. If you are concerned about the raw egg risk of salmonella, buy organic pastured eggs. You can also wash your pastured eggs thoroughly in warm, soapy water before cracking them open. If an egg is contaminated with salmonella, it is usually on the shell, not inside the egg.

1 egg
1 tablespoon Dijon mustard
¾ cup olive oil

2 tablespoons freshly squeezed lemon juice
Sea salt
Freshly ground black pepper

1. In a large bowl, whisk the egg and mustard together until very well combined, about 2 minutes.
2. While whisking, add the olive oil in a continuous thin stream until the mayonnaise is thick and completely emulsified.
3. Whisk in the lemon juice.
4. Season with salt and pepper.
5. Keep in the refrigerator in an airtight container for up to 4 days.

Make It Easy: Mayonnaise is an emulsion, which means whipping two liquids that usually do not mix to form a uniform suspension. Create interesting varieties by stirring in curry powder, horseradish, roasted garlic, roasted red pepper, pesto, or chili powder.

Per Serving (1 tablespoon)
Macronutrients: Fat: 100 percent; Protein: 0 percent; Carbs: 0 percent
Ketogenic Ratio: 5:1
Calories: 48; Total Fat: 5g; Total Carbohydrates: 0g; Fiber: 0g;
Net Carbs: 0g; Protein: <1g; Sugar Alcohols: 0g

Lime Guacamole

SERVES 6 / PREP TIME: 15 MINUTES

Guacamole is a spectacular keto condiment because it can help add fat and flavor to anything you serve it with or on. Fish, chicken, meats, vegetables, and even eggs taste wonderful with rich lime-spiked avocado. The lime will help prevent unsightly oxidization of the avocado, so do not leave it out or you will have an unappetizing gray mush.

2 ripe avocados, peeled and halved
¼ cup finely chopped red onion
2 tablespoons chopped fresh cilantro
1 tablespoon minced jalapeño pepper

1 tablespoon olive oil
1 teaspoon minced garlic
Juice and zest of 1 lime
Sea salt

1. Place the avocado halves in a bowl and mash them with a fork until you have a chunky paste.
2. Stir in the onion, cilantro, jalapeño, olive oil, garlic, lime juice, and lime zest.
3. Season with salt.
4. Store the guacamole in the refrigerator in a sealed container for up to 5 days.

Nutrition Tip: Avocado is high in healthy fats, potassium, and magnesium as well as blood-sugar-stabilizing fiber.

Per Serving
Macronutrients: Fat: 81 percent; Protein: 3 percent; Carbs: 16 percent
Ketogenic Ratio: 3.7:1
Calories: 122; Total Fat: 11g; Total Carbohydrates: 6g; Fiber: 4g;
Net Carbs: 2g; Protein: 1g; Sugar Alcohols: 0g

Chicken Bone Broth

MAKES 8 CUPS / PREP TIME: 15 MINUTES / COOK TIME: 4 TO 6 HOURS

Chicken broth is a tried-and-true method to cure all that ails you.
Remember to save the carcasses of your roasted chickens in
sealed plastic bags in the freezer so you can make batches of this
healthy broth.

2 chicken carcasses

3 celery stalks, cut into 1-inch chunks

2 carrots, peeled and roughly chopped

1 onion, cut into quarters

2 tablespoons apple cider vinegar

4 fresh thyme sprigs

2 fresh bay leaves

Water

1. Preheat the oven to 350°F.
2. Place the chicken carcasses in a baking pan and roast them for 30 minutes.
3. Transfer the carcasses to a large stockpot and add the celery, carrots, onion, vinegar, thyme, bay leaves, and enough water to cover the ingredients by 3 inches.
4. Place the stockpot on high heat and bring to a boil.
5. Reduce the heat to low and gently simmer the broth, partially covered, stirring every few hours, for 4 to 6 hours.
6. Remove the pot from the heat and cool for 15 minutes.
7. Remove the large chicken bones with tongs, then strain the broth through a fine-mesh sieve and discard the solid bits.
8. Pour the stock into containers or jars and cool it completely.
9. Store the stock in sealed containers or jars in the refrigerator for up to 5 days, or in the freezer for up to 3 months.

Per Serving (1 cup)

Macronutrients: Fat: 22 percent; Protein: 78 percent; Carbs: 0 percent

Ketogenic Ratio: 1: 8

Calories: 40; Total Fat: 1g; Total Carbohydrates: 0g; Fiber: 0g;

Net Carbs: 0g; Protein: 8g; Sugar Alcohols: 0g

Beef Bone Broth

MAKES 8 CUPS / PREP TIME: 15 MINUTES / COOK TIME: 7 HOURS

Bone broth has been used for centuries in Chinese medicine to strengthen digestion and the kidneys. In the 12th century, it was prescribed by physicians to cure ailments ranging from the common cold to stomach upsets.

2 pounds beef bones
3 celery stalks, cut into chunks
3 garlic cloves, lightly crushed
2 carrots, peeled and cut into 1-inch chunks

1 onion, cut into quarters
2 tablespoons apple cider vinegar
½ teaspoon whole black peppercorns
Water

1. Preheat the oven to 350°F.
2. Place the beef bones in a deep baking pan and roast them in the oven for 45 minutes.
3. Transfer the roasted bones to a large stockpot and add the celery, garlic, carrots, onion, vinegar, peppercorns, and enough water to cover all the ingredients by about 3 inches.
4. Place the stockpot on high heat and bring to a boil.
5. Reduce the heat to low and simmer the broth, partially covered, for 4 to 6 hours.
6. Check the broth every half hour for the first 2 hours to skim off the foam (impurities) from the top with a spoon.
7. Remove the stockpot from the heat and cool for 15 to 20 minutes.
8. Remove the large beef bones with tongs, then strain the broth through a fine-mesh sieve and discard the solid bits.
9. Pour the stock into containers or jars and allow it to cool completely.
10. Store the stock in sealed containers or jars in the refrigerator for up to 5 days, or in the freezer for up to 3 months.

Per Serving (1 cup)
Macronutrients: Fat: 31 percent; Protein: 69 percent; Carbs: 0 percent
Ketogenic Ratio: 1:5
Calories: 29; Total Fat: 1g; Total Carbohydrates: 0g; Fiber: 0g;
Net Carbs: 0g; Protein: 5g; Sugar Alcohols: 0g

Tips for Dining Out

It's best to keep it simple when dining out. Look for a whole protein, not a casserole or mixed dish (unless it's fajitas, yum!). Next, find a low-carbohydrate vegetable—it could be anything from broccoli to spaghetti squash. The main vegetables to avoid are potatoes and sweet potatoes, but you should also stay away from corn and peas, as these are quite high in carbs. Put a generous serving of butter on your veggies. For salads, leave croutons and tortilla strips off, and use lots of dressing. Choose oil and vinegar, ranch, Italian, or something high-fat but not sweet.

Keep your portions small. In general, 3 ounces of meat is plenty. You may want more than that, but don't. Excess protein will convert to glucose, raise blood sugar, and decrease ketones. You may be served a large pile of vegetables and a generous salad, but it's okay to only eat half. If you are eating lots of fat, you will be satisfied.

Some restaurants are offering keto options now. This is great, usually, if you're aware of what ingredients they're using. Ask a few questions. Sometimes foods like keto pizza or keto tacos are fairly low-carb but quite high in protein, not high-fat, and lacking in vegetables. Foods like that may drop you out of ketosis. Think about eating a half portion of a restaurant keto meal and adding 1 to 2 tablespoons of fat. You may be able to use ranch dressing on the pizza or add oil to the taco.

Here's another thought if you're worried about finding the right foods: There is no rule that you have to eat when out with friends or family. You can eat before or after you go out. You can be social over a club soda or lemon water.

It will help to tell the people closest to you about the changes that you are making. They may not cook a separate meal for you, but they might be willing to cook your chicken with spices instead of barbecue sauce or serve broccoli instead of corn. For family meals, you could offer to bring a dish from one of the tasty recipes in this book. Your family will be glad to see that you're eating healthy foods. Many people don't understand that eating a lower-carb diet can still mean great-tasting meals.

The Dirty Dozen and the Clean Fifteen™

A nonprofit environmental watchdog organization called Environmental Working Group (EWG) looks at data about pesticide residues supplied by the United States Department of Agriculture (USDA) and the Food and Drug Administration (FDA). Each year it compiles a list of the best and worst pesticide loads found in commercial crops. You can use these lists to decide which fruits and vegetables to buy organic to minimize your exposure to pesticides and which produce is considered safe enough to buy conventionally. This does not mean they are pesticide-free, though, so wash these fruits and vegetables thoroughly. The list is updated annually, and you can find it online at EWG.org/FoodNews.

DIRTY DOZEN™

1. strawberries
2. spinach
3. kale
4. nectarines
5. apples
6. grapes
7. peaches
8. cherries
9. pears
10. tomatoes
11. celery
12. potatoes

CLEAN FIFTEEN™

1. avocados
2. sweet corn
3. pineapples
4. sweet peas (frozen)
5. onions
6. papayas
7. eggplants
8. asparagus
9. kiwis
10. cabbages
11. cauliflower
12. cantaloupes
13. broccoli
14. mushrooms
15. honeydew melons

Additionally, nearly three-quarters of hot pepper samples contained pesticide residues.

Measurement Conversions

VOLUME EQUIVALENTS (LIQUID)

US Standard	US Standard (ounces)	Metric (approximate)
2 tablespoons	1 fl. oz.	30 mL
¼ cup	2 fl. oz.	60 mL
½ cup	4 fl. oz.	120 mL
1 cup	8 fl. oz.	240 mL
1½ cups	12 fl. oz.	355 mL
2 cups or 1 pint	16 fl. oz.	475 mL
4 cups or 1 quart	32 fl. oz.	1 L
1 gallon	128 fl. oz.	4 L

OVEN TEMPERATURES

Fahrenheit (F)	Celsius (C) (approximate)
250°F	120°C
300°F	150°C
325°F	165°C
350°F	180°C
375°F	190°C
400°F	200°C
425°F	220°C
450°F	230°C

VOLUME EQUIVALENTS (DRY)

US Standard	Metric (approximate)
⅛ teaspoon	0.5 mL
¼ teaspoon	1 mL
½ teaspoon	2 mL
¾ teaspoon	4 mL
1 teaspoon	5 mL
1 tablespoon	15 mL
¼ cup	59 mL
⅓ cup	79 mL
½ cup	118 mL
⅔ cup	156 mL
¾ cup	177 mL
1 cup	235 mL
2 cups or 1 pint	475 mL
3 cups	700 mL
4 cups or 1 quart	1 L

WEIGHT EQUIVALENTS

US Standard	Metric (approximate)
½ ounce	15 g
1 ounce	30 g
2 ounces	60 g
4 ounces	115 g
8 ounces	225 g
12 ounces	340 g
16 ounces or 1 pound	455 g

Resources

....

MCT OIL

MCT (medium-chain triglyceride) oil is commonly used in ketogenic diet plans. It will raise ketones better than other fats, so it's a fantastic addition to your diet. Don't be afraid to use a significant amount of MCT oil (up to 25 percent of your calories), but work up to it gradually to avoid gastrointestinal problems such as nausea, vomiting, and diarrhea. Many people start out with 1 tablespoon per day and work up to 3 to 4 tablespoons a day over the course of a month with no ill effects. Spread it throughout the day and count it as part of the fat needed in your meals. Remember, this is optional but helpful for increasing ketones.

HOW TO MEASURE KETOSIS

To know whether you are achieving therapeutic ketosis, it's best to measure your blood ketones. You may do this by purchasing a blood glucose meter that also measures ketones. It uses one strip for glucose and a different strip for ketones. Nutritional ketosis is commonly considered to be ketones greater than 0.5mmol/L. You may need ketones much higher than this to stop your migraines. Ketosis of 1.0–4.0mmol/L would be a good goal. When you use a meter, you will see the impact different meals and foods have on ketones and can make adjustments accordingly.

You may also get strips that check urine ketones, to get a rough idea of whether or not your body has adapted to burning fat for energy (achieved ketosis). Urine measurements are affected by hydration status, time of day, and the integrity of the strip. Urine testing is quite inexpensive, but blood testing will give you more specific information to work with as you adapt and make dietary adjustments.

Two common brands of blood ketone/glucose meters are:

Precision Xtra by Abbott: abbottstore.com/precision-xtra-blood-glucose-ketone-monitoring-system-1-pack-9881465.html

Keto Mojo by Keto Mojo: keto-mojo.com

HELPFUL TOOLS AND INFORMATION

MIND AND BODY

Self Magazine 21 Best Stretching Exercises for Better Flexibility: www.self.com/gallery/essential-stretches-slideshow

Great pictures and directions for 21 essential stretches to round out any fitness routine.

Mindful: www.mindful.org/how-to-meditate/

Mindful.org is a stellar resource on mindfulness and meditation and helps you understand pain, decrease stress, improve focus, and more with practical steps and guidance.

FOOD TRACKER APPS

My Fitness Pal: www.myfitnesspal.com

Track macros and exercise and meet personal goals with this free, easy-to-use online food tracking app.

Cronometer: cronometer.com

Cronometer is an excellent app for those who would like to track macros, nutrients, ketone readings, and fitness in a very detailed fashion.

Carb Manager: www.carbmanager.com

A lovely, user-friendly app to track your macros, find new recipes, and see data in a well-organized, aesthetically appealing way.

KETOGENIC DIET WEBSITES

The Charlie Foundation: charliefoundation.org

The Charlie Foundation for Ketogenic Diet Therapies (KDT) was founded in 1994 to provide information about diet therapies for people with epilepsy, other neurological disorders, and certain cancers. The Charlie Foundation is one of the oldest and most trusted KDT resources.

Matthew's Friends: www.matthewsfriends.org

Matthew's Friends supports patients, families, and professionals by providing information, training, research, and grants to develop ketogenic services and support systems for epilepsy and other neurological disorders, as well as emerging cancer types.

Epilepsy Foundation: www.epilepsy.com

The mission of the Epilepsy Foundation is to lead the fight to overcome the challenges of living with epilepsy and to accelerate therapies to stop seizures, find cures, and save lives.

KetoDietCalculator: www.ketodietcalculator.org

KetoDietCalculator is a web-based program provided by the Charlie Foundation to manage therapeutic ketogenic diets. Certified clinicians are given an account to which they add individual clients. The clients are given access to the program to plan meals according to clinician recommendations. The program assists with meal, snack, and fluid calculations, supplement analysis, medication review, and has an expandable database.

References

....

American Headache Society. "Opioids and migraine." Accessed July 1, 2019. https://americanheadachesociety.org/news/opioids-migraine/.

American Migraine Foundation. "The timeline of a migraine attack." Published January 18, 2018. https://americanmigrainefoundation.org/resource-library/timeline-migraine-attack/.

Association of Migraine Disorders. "Cognitive-behavioral therapy (CBT) is a psychological approach to managing headaches and migraine." Published March 30, 2018. https://www.migrainedisorders.org/why-try-cognitive-behavioral-therapy-for-migraine/.

Barbanti, et al. "Ketogenic diet in migraine: rationale, findings, and perspectives." *Neurological Sciences* 38, supplement 1 (2017): S111–S115.

Brenton, et al. "Pilot study of a ketogenic diet in relapsing-remitting MS." *Neurology, Neuroimmunology & Neuroinflammation* 6, no. 4 (July, 2019): https://doi.org/10.1212/NXI.0000000000000565.

DiLorenzo, et al. "Diet transiently improves migraines in two twin sisters: possible role of ketogenesis?" *Functional Neurology* 28, no. 4 (October–December 2013): https://www.ncbi.nlm.nih.gov/pmc/articles/PMC3951260/.

DiLorenzo, et al. "Migraine improvement during short lasting ketogenesis: a proof-of-concept study." *European Journal of Neurology* 22, no. 1 (January 2015): doi:10.1111/ene.12550.

DiLorenzo, et al. "Cortical functional correlates of responsiveness to short-lasting preventative intervention with ketogenic diet in migraine: a multimodal evoked potentials study." *The Journal of Headache and Pain* 17, no. 58 (May 2016): doi:10.1186/s10194-016-0650-9.

Goadsby, et al. "Pathophysiology of migraine: a disorder of sensory processing." *Physiological Reviews* 97, no. 2 (April 2017): doi:10.1152/physrev.00034.2015.

Hajihashemi, et al. "The effects of concurrent Coenzyme Q10, L-carnitine supplementation in migraine prophylaxis: a randomized, placebo-controlled, double-blind trial." *Cephalalgia* 39, no. 5 (April 2019): doi: 10.1177/0333102418821661.

Hernandez-Reif, et al. "Migraine headaches are reduced by massage therapy." *International Journal of Neuroscience* 96, no. 1–2 (March 1998): https://doi.org/10.3109/00207459808986453.

Jackson, et al. "Botulinum toxin A for prophylactic treatment of migraine and tension head-aches in adults: a meta-analysis." *Journal of the American Medical Association* 307, no. 16 (April 25, 2012): doi:10.1001/jama.2012.505.

Kılıç, B., and Kılıç, M. "Evaluation of vitamin D levels and response to therapy of childhood migraine." *Medicina (Kaunas)* 55, no. 7 (June 2019): doi:10.3390/medicina55070321.

Kossoff, et al. *The Ketogenic and Modified Atkins Diets*, 6th Edition. New York: Demos Health, 2016.

Linde, et al. "Acupuncture for migraine prophylaxis." *Cochrane Database of Systematic Reviews* (January 21, 2009): doi:10.1002/14651858.CD001218.pub2.

Moore, et al. "A critical review of manual therapy use for headache disorders: prevalence, profiles, motivations, communication and self-reported effectiveness." *BMC Neurology* 17, no. 1 (March 2017): doi:10.1186/s12883-017-0835-0.

Moscano, et al. "An observational study of fixed dose *Tanacetum parthenium* nutraceutical preparation for prophylaxis of pediatric headache." *Italian Journal of Pediatrics* 45, no. 36 (2019): doi:10.1186/s13052-019-0624-z.

Napoli, et al. "Potential therapeutic use of the ketogenic diet in autism spectrum disorders." *Frontiers in Pediatrics* 2 (June 2014): doi:10.3389/fped.2014.00069.

Niemiec, R. "Three definitions of mindfulness that might surprise you." Published November 1, 2017. https://www.psychologytoday.com/us/blog/what-matters-most/201711/3 -definitions-mindfulness-might-surprise-you.

Pardutz, A., and Schoenen, J. "NSAIDs in the acute treatment of migraine; a review of clinical and experimental data." *Pharmaceuticals (Basel)* 3, no. 6 (June 2010): doi:10.3390/ph3061966.

Parohan, et al. "The synergistic effects of nano-curcumin and coenzyme Q10 supplementation in migraine prophylaxis: a randomized, placebo-controlled, double-blind trial." *Nutritional Neuroscience* (June 2019): doi:10.1080/1028415x.2019.1627770.

Seyfried, et al. "Provocative question: should ketogenic metabolic therapy become the standard of care for glioblastoma?" *Neurochemical Research* (April 2019): doi:10.1007 /s11064-019-02795-4.

Trinh, et al. "Systematic review of episodic migraine prophylaxis: efficacy of conventional treatments used in comparisons with acupuncture." *Medical Acupuncture* 31, no. 2 (April 2019): doi:10.1089/acu.2019.1337.

Vanitallie, et al. "Treatment of Parkinson disease with diet-induced hyperketonemia: a feasibility study." *Neurology* 64, no. 4 (February 2005): doi:10.1212/01.WNL.0000152046.11390.45.

Varkey, et al. "Exercise as migraine prophylaxis: a randomized study using relaxation and topiramate as controls." *Cephalgia* 31, no. 14 (September 2011): doi:10.1177/0333102411419681.

Viana, et al. "Clinical features of visual migraine aura: a systematic review." *The Journal of Headache and Pain* 20, no. 64 (May 2019): doi:10.1186/s10194-019-1008-x.

WebMD. "TMS as a treatment for migraine headaches." Published May 19, 2019. https://www.webmd.com/migraines-headaches/tms-for-migraines#1.

Winter, et al. "Role of ketogenic metabolic therapy in malignant glioma: a systematic review." *Critical Reviews in Oncology/Hematology* 112 (February 2017): doi:10.1016/j.critrevonc.2017.02.016.

Wlodarek, D. "Role of ketogenic diets in neurodegenerative diseases (Alzheimer's disease and Parkinson's disease)." *Nutrients* 11, no. 1 (January 2019): doi:10.3390/nu11010169.

Zimetbaum, P. "5 Migraine Questions Answered." Harvard Health Publishing. Accessed September 13, 2019. https://health.harvard.edu/healthbeat/5-migraine-questions-answered.

Zuccoli, et al. "Metabolic management of glioblastoma multiforme using standard therapy together with a restricted ketogenic diet: Case Report." *Nutrition & Metabolism* 7, no. 33 (April 2010): doi:10.1186/1743-7075-7-33.

Index

Acknowledgments

So many people contributed to my growth and success as a keto dietitian: Beth Zupec-Kania, who mentored me from my start in the area more than 12 years ago; the excellent keto team at CS Mott Children's Hospital (University of Michigan); my many conference buddies (you know who you are!); the awesome keto parents who sometimes taught me as much as I taught them; the keto kids, who smiled and learned and grew on only a few carbs (who knew? . . . we did!); and the brave adults who are using this diet for numerous medical conditions, successfully paving the way for others.

Thank you to Jim and Nancy Abrahams for founding The Charlie Foundation for Ketogenic Therapies 25 years ago and sparking a crusade that has changed the world.

I am forever grateful to my parents for raising me to believe I was capable of achieving anything I was willing to work for.

I am so thankful for a supportive husband who encourages me to live out my dreams, and I am also amazed at my four wonderful kids—two adults and two at home. I am blessed. They each see life differently, but I think they all get it.

I thank God for life and breath and sustenance, and for creating our bodies in such a way that many problems can be healed with healthy, wholesome foods.

And thank you, butter—together we will defeat migraines, epilepsy, cancer, Parkinson's, ALS, MS, and many other conditions . . . one stick at a time.